ENDOSCOPIC PROCEDURES IN COLON AND RECTUM

Edited by **José Joaquim Ribeiro da Rocha**

Endoscopic Procedures in Colon and Rectum
Edited by José Joaquim Ribeiro da Rocha

Published by InTech
Janeza Trdine 9, 51000 Rijeka, Croatia

Publishing Process Manager Igor Babic

Technical Editor Teodora Smiljanic

Cover Designer InTech Design Team

Additional hard copies can be obtained from orders@intechopen.com

Endoscopic Procedures in Colon and Rectum, Edited by José Joaquim Ribeiro da Rocha
p. cm.
ISBN 978-953-307-677-5

Meet the editor

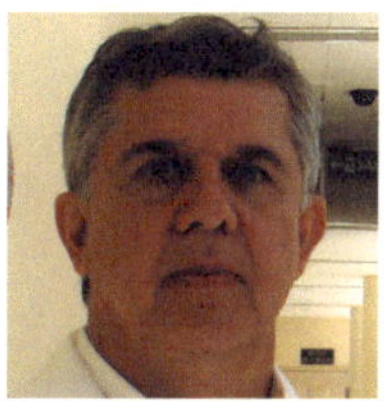

Dr. José Joaquim Ribeiro da Rocha is a professor of surgery in the area of Coloproctology in Brazil, University of São Paulo, Faculty of Medicine of Ribeirão Preto. He has made research in diffuse peritonitis, intestinal anastomosis and transanal endoscopic operations. He has also been directing the Division of Coloproctology at the Faculty of Medicine of Ribeirão Preto - University of São Paulo since 2004. He is editor of the book "Coloproctology - Principles and Practices", edited by Atheneu publishing house, now in 2011 in its second edition. He earned his master and PhD degrees in surgery at the Department of Surgery and Anatomy of the Faculty of Medicine of Ribeirão Preto – University of São Paulo – Brazil. He is also a coloproctology surgeon at the Hospital São Paulo – Ribeirão Preto – State of São Paulo – Brazil.

Contents

Preface

Coloproctology has made tremendous progress, asserting itself as a specialty, it has been taught in all medical schools and chosen by many as an option in their careers. There are numerous textbooks that discuss in detail the various issues of Coloproctology. In this age of computers and virtual reality, when the knowledge they accumulate and recycle increases each day dramatically, one would be able to question the decision to make another book on this subject.

When I was invited to edit this publication, I felt as a challenge to review and compile the chapters presented in this work and make it appropriate and useful to those who will consult it.

The chapters of screening and surveillance, preparation, monitoring and considerations about intestinal inflammation through colonoscopy, lead us to current knowledge and accurate guidance in the improvement of those who already performs colonoscopies and those who wish to develop research or improve clinical performance.

The studies of virtual colonoscopy, intraoperative enteroscopy, transanal endoscopic operations and the treatment of rectal varices show the quality of the experts in diagnosing and treating ailments with accuracy, the lessons that challenge the knowledge and the technical skills possessed by the endoscopists and surgeons of today.

It is a different book, nice and easy to read. Its nine chapters were written by authors from many different countries, are well designed and they exhaust the subject within their themes. I am extremely honored to preface and edit this book and I congratulate all the authors on their work.

José Joaquim Ribeiro da Rocha
Division of Coloproctology of the Department of Surgery and Anatomy,
Ribeirão Preto Faculty of Medicine – University of São Paulo
Brazil

1

Screening and Surveillance Colonoscopy

Miroslav Zavoral[1], Stepan Suchanek[1], Ondrej Majek[2], Barbora Rotnaglova[1] and Jan Martinek[1]

[1]*Charles University, 1st Medical Faculty, Central Military Hospital, Department of Medicine, Prague*

[2]*Masaryk University, Institute of Biostatistics and Analyses, Brno*

Czech Republic

1. Introduction

Colorectal cancer (CRC) is the second most frequent malignant disease in Europe. Every year, 412,000 people are diagnosed with this condition, and 207,000 patients die of it. Secondary prevention of CRC consists of early diagnosis of the disease in asymptomatic individuals (screening) and long term follow up of high risk patients (surveillance). Three groups of screening methods are currently available: stool testing (guaiac or immunochemical fecal occult blood tests - gFOBT and FIT respectively and DNA tests), endoscopic examinations (flexible sigmoidoscopy and colonoscopy) and radiologic examinations (computed tomographic colonography and double contrast barium enema). Colonoscopy is therefore used as the only screening method or as a second step in case of positive results of primary screening examination (two steps screening programs). From 27 countries in the European Union, the most frequently used test is FOBT (in 11 states). There is a choice between FOBT and colonoscopy in 6 countries. FOBT and flexible sigmoidoscopy is available in Italy. Currently, the only country using colonoscopy as the only screening method is Poland. At the end of 2010, the European guidelines for quality assurance in colorectal cancer screening and diagnosis were published, summarizing the evidence based medicine data for the efficacy, the interval, the age range, the risk-benefit and cost-effectiveness of colonoscopy screening. Unfortunately, prospective randomized trial on the effect of screening colonoscopy in the reduction of CRC incidence and mortality has not been published yet. Promising should be the NordICC study, which was introduced in 2009, however the results will be available in a fifteen year period. Series of recently published studies (Canada, Germany, Poland) focusing on the interval (post-colonoscopic) cancers confirmed the inadequate protection of proximal colon by colonoscopy. Another important issue would be the quality and safety of colonoscopy and the bowel cleansing. Concerning the surveillance colonoscopy, it plays a major role in specific follow up strategies in CRC high risk groups. It can be concluded that with some limitations, colonoscopy still remains the fundamental diagnostic and prophylactic examination in colorectal cancer screening and surveillance.

2. Colorectal cancer epidemiology in Europe

Colorectal cancer is the second most frequent malignant disease in developed countries. CRC incidence is generally higher in male population, and the risk of the disease increases with age, as the majority of cases are diagnosed in patients over 50 years of age (Spann et al., 2002). Burden of European countries is ranked as the highest in the global statistics, both in incidence and mortality. Compared to the US, in 1998 - 2002 the European population showed a similar incidence for men, while that for women was slightly lower; the incidence in the USA for men and women was 38.6 and 28.3 respectively: in Europe it was 38.5 and 24.6 (ASR-W), as calculated per 100,000 inhabitants (Curado et al., 2007) . However, mortality over the same period of time was significantly higher in Europe than in the US, both for men and women: in the USA the figures were 13.5 and 9.2 respectively, while in Europe they were 18.5 and 10.7 (ASR-W), as calculated per 100,000 inhabitants (World Health Organization [WHO], 2006). To document the situation in Europe, we used figures available from the international studies summarizing global and European epidemiologic data (Curado et al., 2007; Ferlay et al., 2004, 2007; Parkin et al., 2005). A detailed comparison of countries within Europe using the global age standardization (ASR-W) of incidence is presented in figure 1.

Incidence in international comparison – European countries

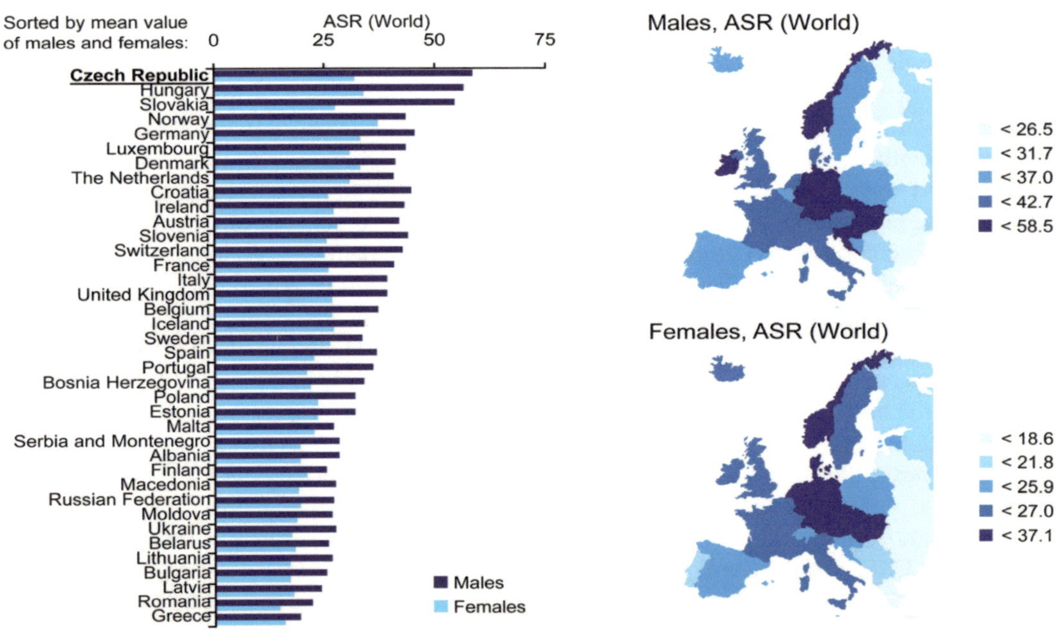

Fig. 1. International comparison of CRC incidence in European countries

Colorectal cancer comprises 12.9% of all newly-diagnosed carcinomas in the European population (men 12.8%, women 13.1%) and account for 12.2% of deaths caused by malignancy. Colorectal cancer is the second most common malignancy, after breast carcinoma (13.5% of all malignities), followed by bronchogenic carcinoma (12.1% of all malignancies). Every year 412,900 people are diagnosed with CRC in Europe, and 207,400 of them die of the disease (Ferlay et al., 2007). The average incidence has shown a tendency to rise in recent years, with an annual increment 0.5%. Data available regarding time trends of CRC mortality are displayed in figure 2. The CRC-related mortality has stabilized or shown a slight decrease over recent years.

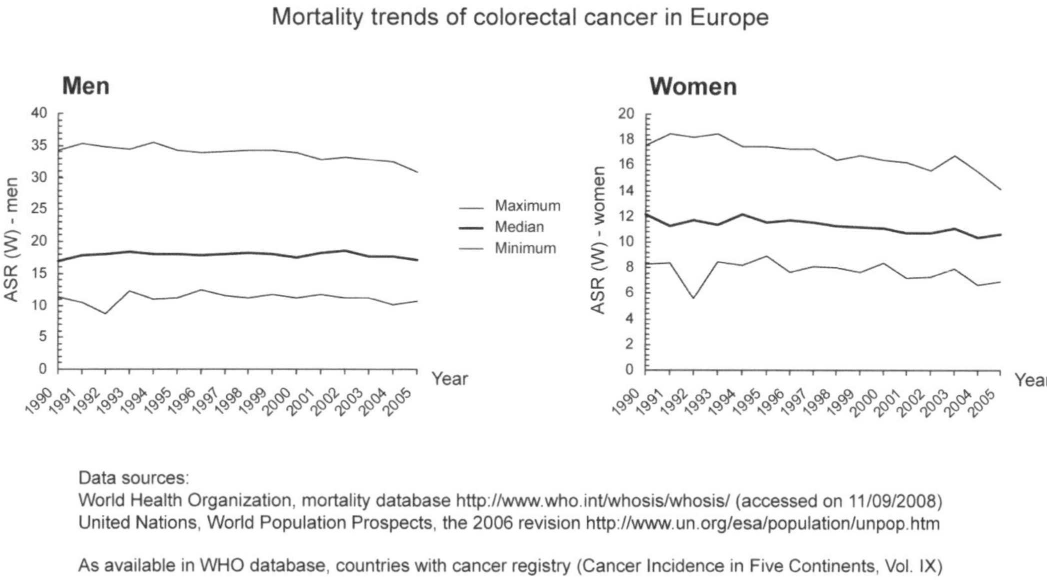

Fig. 2. Colorectal cancer mortality trends in Europe (men left, women right)

3. Colorectal cancer prevention

Colorectal cancer belongs to preventable cancers. Primary prevention focuses on dietary and lifestyle recommendations. Secondary prevention of CRC consists of early diagnosis of the disease in asymptomatic individuals (screening) in patients older than 50 years of age and a long term follow up of high risk patients (surveillance).

4. Colorectal cancer screening

Three groups of screening methods are currently available (see in the table below): stool testing (guaiac or immunochemical fecal occult blood tests – gFOBT and FIT respectively and DNA tests), endoscopic examinations (flexible sigmoidoscopy and colonoscopy) and radiologic examinations (computed tomographic colonography and double contrast barium enema). Colonoscopy is therefore used as the only screening method or as a second step in case of positive results of primary screening examination (Zavoral et al, 2009).

Type of method	Method
Stool tests	for presence of occult blood
	guaiac-based (gFOBT)
	immunochemical (FIT)
	for presence of abnormal DNA
Endoscopic examinations	flexible sigmoideoscopy (FS)
	colonoscopy
Radiologic examinations	computed tomographic colonography (CTC)
	double contrast barium enema (DCBE)

Table 1. Overview of CRC screening methods

In 2008, the Report on the Implementation of the Council Recommendation on Cancer Screening, which provides the most comprehensive data available, was published (Karsa et al., 2008). According to this report, CRC screening is running or being established in 19 of 27 EU countries. The target group contains approximately 136 million individuals suitable for CRC screening (aged 50 to 74 years). Of this number, 43% individuals come from 12 countries where CRC population screening is performed or being prepared on either national or regional levels; 34% come from 5 countries where national population screening has been implemented (Finland, France, Italy, Poland, and United Kingdom). In 7 EU countries, national non-population based screening is carried out, which covers 27% of the target population. In 2007, gFOBT (which was the only test recommended by the Council of the European Union in 2003) was used as the only screening method in twelve countries (Bulgaria, Czech Republic, Finland, France, Hungary, Latvia, Portugal, Romania, Slovenia, Spain, Sweden, and United Kingdom). Colonoscopy was the only screening method used in Poland. In six countries, two types of tests were used: iFOBT and FS in Italy, and gFOBT and colonoscopy in Austria, Cyprus, Germany, Greece, and Slovak Republic. In the remaining eight states (Belgium, Denmark, Estonia, Ireland, Lithuania, Luxembourg, Malta, and the Netherlands), CRC screening has not been implemented yet. The age limit for the target population varies across the EU countries. In 2007, it was estimated that a total of 12 million individuals participated in CRC screening.

4.1 Selected colonoscopy CRC screening programs

Poland is currently the only state using colonoscopy as the only screening method, without the alternative of FOBT. An opportunistic screening programme was initiated in 2000, and by now, this had grown to 80 centers across the whole of Poland. The programme is financed by the Ministry of Health, independentantly from the overall healthcare system. The target population (asymptomatic individuals aged 55–66 years) is recruited through general practitioners. High emphasis is placed on the quality control of colonoscopies, with complications reported for 0.1% procedures, and no patient dying. The advantage of the programme consists in thorough monitoring and evaluation, including monitoring of interval cancers (Regula et al., 2006).

Germany was the first country to introduce a population screening programme (in 1976) based on an annual gFOBT for individuals older than 44 years of age. Starting in 2002, the participants were offered a choice between colonoscopy at 55 years of age (in a ten-year interval) and FOBT in annual intervals between 50 and 54 years of age and in a two-year interval after 55 years of age. In case of FOBT positivity, screening colonoscopy followed. Between 2003 - 2008, there were 2 821 392 colonoscopies performed in over 2 100 practices all over Germany. The cumulative participation rate was 17.2% for women and 15.5% for men. Adenomas were diagnosed in a total of 19.4%, advanced adenomas in 6.4% and carcinomas in 0.9% of the examined patients. The majority of cancers were in early stage (UICC 47.3%, UICC II 22.3%, UICC III 20.7%, and UICC IV 9.6%). The overall and serious complication rate was 2.8 and 0.58 respectively per 1 000 colonoscopies. The cost analyses have proven the cost effectiveness of such screening (Pox et al., 2007).

In the Czech Republic, CRC screening has many years of tradition. It was the second country in the world to start a nation-wide screening programme (in 2000), based on biennial gFOBT offered to asymptomatic individuals older than 50 years of age. In order to achieve higher compliance rate, screening colonoscopy was added to current FOBT screening as an alternative method in 2009, in the same intervals as in the German programme. Both, gFOBT and various types of FIT are offered as well. During years 2006 - 2010, there were 47 760 screening colonoscopies (FOBT+) and 5 574 primary screening colonoscopies performed. Adenomas and carcinomas were diagnosed in 16 454 (30.9%) and 2 539 (4.8%) respectively. The proportion of advanced adenomas and generalized cancer (UICC stage III and IV) was 48% and 20.7% respectively (Zavoral et al., 2009).

4.2 Screening colonoscopy studies

The multinational NordICC (The Nordic-European Initiative on Colorectal Cancer) study was introduced in June 2009, however the results will be available in a fifteen year period. This study focuses on monitoring the effect of colonoscopy screening on reducing CRC incidence and mortality. The northern states of Europe (Norway, Sweden, and Iceland), Poland, and the Netherlands all participate. The Czech Republic, Hungary and Latvia are currently observers and may join the study later. According to the study protocol, a minimum of 66,000 individuals aged 55 to 64 years will be drawn directly from population registers in the participating countries and randomly assigned to either once-only colonoscopy screening or no screening (2:1 randomization, men and women). The primary objective is to compare the incidence and mortality against the control group after 15 years. At this time, more than 5 500 individuals have been examined so far and the recruitment will continue until the end of 2012 (NordiCC Study Protocol, 2011).

CONFIRM (Colonoscopy vs. Fecal Immunochemical Test Reducing Mortality from Colorectal Cancer), the VA Cooperative study, is a multicenter, randomized, parallel group trial directly comparing screening colonoscopy with annual FIT screening in average risk individuals. The quantitative FIT (OC Sensor Diana) cut-off will be set at 100 ng/ml. The primary endpoint expected is CRC mortality reduction by 40% within a 10 year enrolment. The planned study duration is 12.5 years with 2.5 years of recruitment of 50 000 participants (1:1 randomization, 95% men, aged 50 - 75) and 2.5 years of follow-up for enrolled participants (Dominitz et al., 2011).

COLONPREV (Colorectal Cancer Screening in Average-Risk Population: a Multicenter, Randomized Controlled Trial Comparing Immunochemical Fecal Occult Blood Testing versus Colonoscopy) study is being carried out since November 2008 in eight Spanish regions under the coordination of the public health system, primary care physicians and tertiary academic medical centers. Asymptomatic individuals aged 50 - 69 years have been randomized into two groups (1:1). Biennial quantitative FIT (OC Sensor, cut-off level 75 ng/ml), followed by colonoscopy in case of its positivity has been offered to one group and colonoscopy to the second group. First preliminary results are expected in June 2011 (Castellas et al., 2011)

The Japan Polyp Study (JPS) is a multicenter randomized control trial focusing on postpolypectomy surveillance and conducted in eleven centers since February 2003. Two complete colonoscopies with the removal of all neoplastic lesions (to reach "clean colon") have been performed to the enrolled patients who have been randomized into two groups (1:1) afterwards, according to the colonoscopy follow-up interval. One group underwent a colonoscopy after 48 months, the second group at 24 and 48 months. From a total of 4 752 individuals, 3 926 (83%) agreed with the initial colonoscopy and 2 757 (58%) patients were randomized. There has been a great impact on polyp distribution and macroscopic type in the first two initial colonoscopies. Very high adenoma detection (63%) was reached (Matsuda, 2011).

4.3 Screening colonoscopy characteristics

At the end of 2010, the European guidelines for quality assurance in colorectal cancer screening and diagnosis were published, summarizing the evidence based medicine data for the efficacy, the interval, the age range, the risk-benefit and cost-effectiveness of colorectal cancer screening, including sigmoidoscopy (FS) and colonoscopy screening analysis.

4.3.1 Evidence for effectiveness of sigmoidoscopy screening

Flexible sigmoidoscopy screening reduces colorectal cancer (CRC) incidence and mortality if performed in an organised screening programme with careful monitoring of the quality and systematic evaluation of the outcomes, adverse effects and costs (Atkin et al., 2010). The evidence on the efficacy is avaible from randomised controlled trials (RCTs). The most important one is the large UK study in which 57 237 individuals were randomised into the screening group for a once-only sigmoidoscopy alone. This study found a significant 31% reduction in CRC mortality and also a significant reduction in CRC incidence from sigmoidoscopy in an intention-to-treat analysis (Atkin et al., 2010).

The optimal interval for sigmoidoscopy screening was only assessed in two indirect studies that only considered intervals of three and five years (Platell et al., 2002, Schoen et al., 2003). The UK flexible sigmoidoscopy screening study showed that there was little attenuation of the protective effect of sigmoidoscopy after 11 years of follow-up. This is in line with the evidence for colonoscopy screening. In conclusion, the optimal interval for endoscopy screening should not be less than 10 years and may even be extended to 20 years (Atkin et al., 2010).

There is limited evidence suggesting that the best age range for flexible sigmoidoscopy screening should be between 55 and 64 years (Segnan et al., 2007). One study demonstrated that elderly subjects (75 years old) have an increased rate of endoscopist-reported difficulties and a higher rate of incomplete examinations compared to subjects aged 50–74 years (Pabby et al, 2005). Average-risk sigmoidoscopy screening should be discontinued after 74 years of age, given the increasing co-morbidity in this age range (Atkin et al., 2010).

4.3.2 Evidence for effectiveness of colonoscopy screening

Limited evidence exists on the efficacy of colonoscopy screening on CRC incidence and mortality (Atkin et al, 2010). However, two recent case–control studies found a significant reduction of 31% in CRC mortality (Baxter et al., 2009) and 48% in advanced neoplasia detection rates (Brenner et al., 2010). The reduction in these studies was limited to the rectum and left side of the colon. No significant reduction was found in right-sided disease. Cross-sectional surveys have shown that colonoscopy is more sensitive than sigmoidoscopy in detecting adenomas and cancers and that this increased sensitivity could translate into increased effectiveness (Walsh et al., 2003). The efficacy of colonoscopy as a primary screening test has not been proven by prospective randomized control trial.

The optimal interval for colonoscopy screening has been assessed in a cohort study and a case-control study. The cohort study found that CRC incidence in a population with negative colonoscopy was 31% lower than general population rates and remained reduced beyond 10 years after the negative colonoscopy (Singh et al., 2006). Similar results were obtained in the case–control study (Brenner et al., 2006) where the reduction of risk of CRC was 74 % and persisted up to 20 years.

Screening colonoscopies do not need to be performed at intervals shorter than 10 years and this time interval may even be extended to 20 years (Atkin et al., 2010).
There is no direct evidence confirming the optimal age range for colonoscopy screening. Indirect evidence suggests that the prevalence of neoplastic lesions in the younger population (less than 50 years) is too low to justify colonoscopic screening, while in the elderly population (more than 75 years) the lack of benefit could be a major issue (Pabby et al., 2005). The optimal age for a single colonoscopy appears to be around 55 years. Average risk colonoscopy screening should not be performed before age 50 and should be discontinued after 74 years of age (Atkin et al., 2010).

5. Colonoscopic surveillance following adenoma removal

The adenomatous polyp is the precursor of most colorectal cancers and is the most frequently detected lesion during a colonoscopy examination (Lieberman et al., 2000). Hyperplastic polyps, on the other hand, usually have no clinical significance. Based on the statistics, in 33 % - 50 % of patients consecutive adenomas develop within three years after the removal of first adenoma. In addition, in 0,3-0,9 % of cases colorectal carcinoma is detected within five years (Alberts et al., 2000; Arber et al., 2006; Baron et al., 2006; Martinez et al., 2009; Robertson et al., 2005). Most of these adenomas and malignancies are, however, represented by lesions missed during the first colonoscopy. The quality of a colonoscopic examination must therefore be emphasized. Medical centers involved in screening programmes thus often undergo quality controls. One of the key aims of a surveillance colonoscopy is to detect all new lesions or lesions that have been missed at baseline colonoscopy before they progress to malignancy. The other aim of a follow-up colonoscopy is the detection of colorectal carcinoma at an early, prognostically more favorable stage (Robertson et al., 2005).

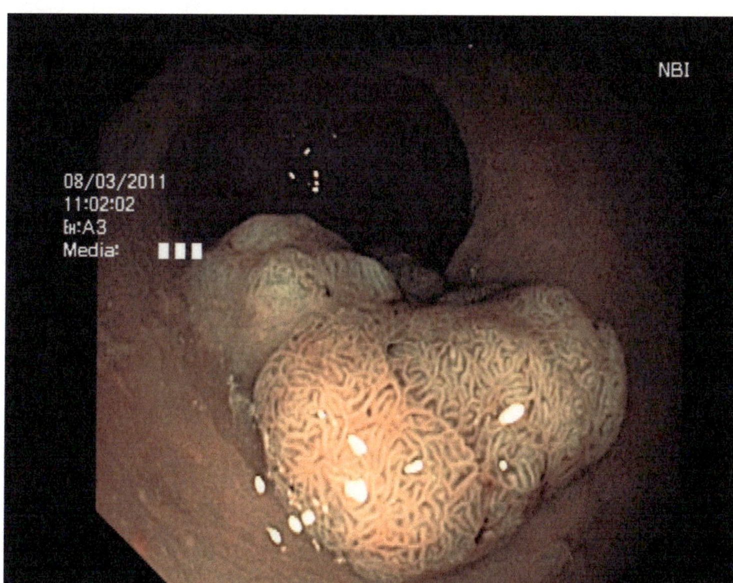

Picture 1. Sessile polyp - white light

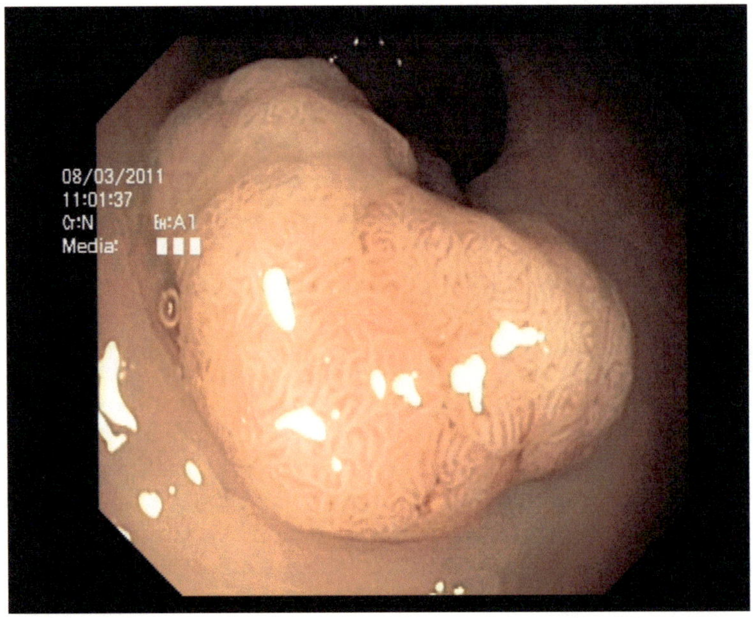

Picture 2. Sessile polyp - NBI (narrow band imaging)

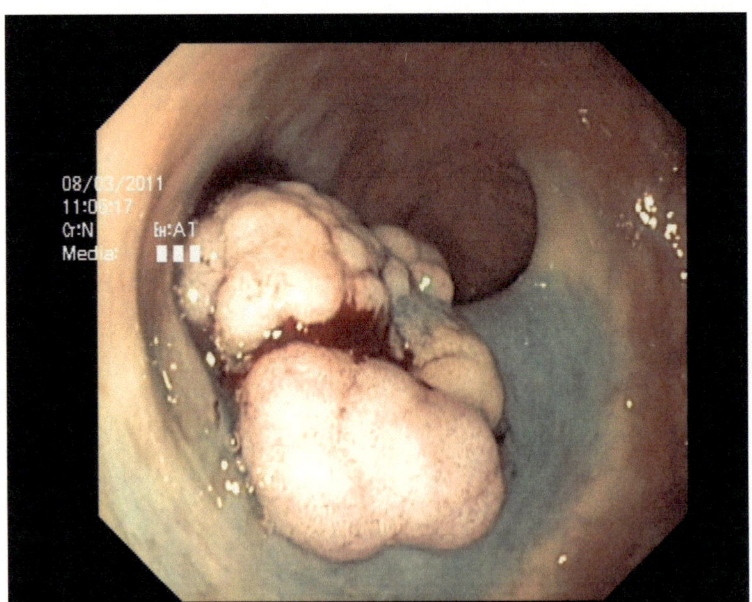

Picture 3. Sessile polyp - Patent Blue injection

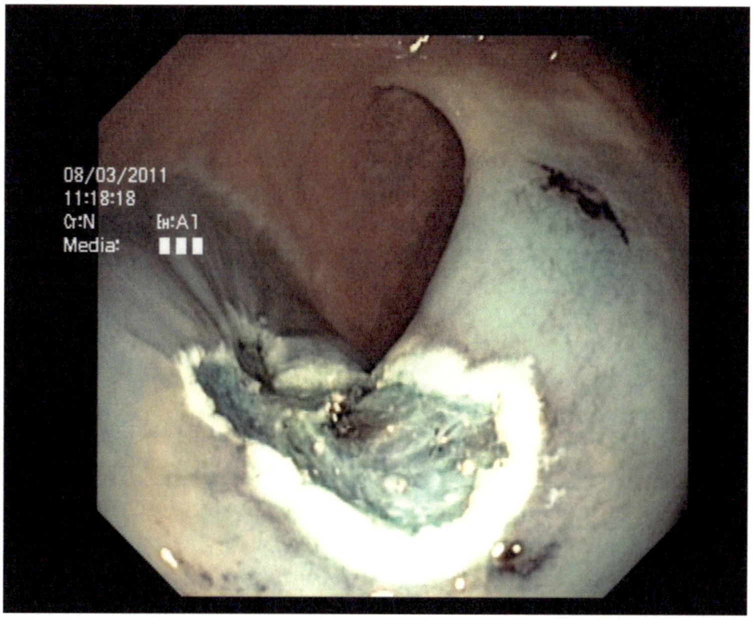

Picture 4. Postpolypectomy site

Colonoscopy is an invasive method with a small, however not insignificant risk of possible complications, amongst which are perforation (0,06 % diagnostic and 2 % therapeutical colonoscopies) and hemorrhage after polypectomy (02,-2,7 % according to size of lesion) (Rosen et al., 1993). Surveillance colonoscopies represent a burden for endoscopic centers prolonging the waiting lists. For these reasons, surveillance colonoscopies should be carried out in recommended intervals in order to prevent the development of colorectal carcinoma. The malignant potential of an adenoma depends on its size, histological verification and the grade of dysplasia. It is higher in advanced adenomas (larger than 10 mm or more, with a villous component or a high grade dysplasia). Recent studies show, that the villous component is a less significant predictor for the development of malignancy than the remaining two factors.

5.1 Risk factors for advanced adenomas and colorectal cancer after baseline polypectomy

The risk of detection of advanced adenoma or carcinoma during a surveillance colonoscopy depends on the quality of the first (baseline) colonoscopy and the characteristics of the removed polyp.

It is generally agreed that high quality colonoscopies carried out less frequently are more efficient in the prevention of colorectal cancer than more frequent colonoscopies of a lower quality. Colonoscopy examination should only be carried out after adequate bowel preparation in order to properly visualize bowel mucosa. Patients with poor bowel preparation have to be invited for a repeated colonoscopy, considering the colonoscopy was well indicated in the first place. The examination must also be complete (reaching the caecum) and the withdrawal of an endoscope should be slow and careful. All detected lesions have to be removed carefully, ideally as hoc during their detection since they can easily be overlooked during the next examination. Polyp removal must be done during the withdrawal of a scope due to the possible risk of bleeding and perforation.

Based on the following meta-analysis (Saini et al., 2006) it is obvious that a personal history of 3 adenomatous polyps increases the risk for the presence of advanced adenoma 2x, whereas the history of five polyps increases the risk at a surveillance colonoscopy 4x, as opposed to the detection of a single polyp during a baseline colonoscopy. The polyp size also plays a significant role. The real size is considered to be the size of the histological specimen measured by a pathologist. In case a piece-meal polypectomy is performed, the size is based upon the judgment of the endoscopist (comparing the lesion with a known size of biopsy forceps). Adenomas measuring between 10 to 20 mm have twice the increased risk, adenomas measuring 20 mm or more have 3x the increased risk of turning to malignancy as opposed to small adenomas (up to 10mm) (Cafferty et al., 2007).

Adenoma histology does not play as significant role as believed earlier. However, a villous structure polyp increases the chance of villous adenoma detection during a surveillance colonoscopy (Cafferty et al., 2007). On the other hand, the presence of high grade dysplasia significantly increases the risk of malignant changes in adenomas of varying size (Saini et al., 2006).

Based on the studies listed below, the localization of polyp in the right colon increases the risk of advanced colorectal neoplasia 1,5-2,5 times as opposed to its localization in the left colon (Laiyemo et al., 2009; Martinez et al., 2009; Saini et al., 2006)

5.2 Risk factors in patients

One of the risk factors is older age, which correlates with the higher incidence of advanced colorectal neoplasia, at the same time it is related to an increased difficulty of a colonoscopy examination and its performance, worse bowel preparation and a higher risk of complications related to the examination itself. It is always necessary to proceed individually recognizing all comorbidities of a patient, the benefit of the examination itself, whilst considering whether the lead time for progression of adenoma to colorectal cancer does not exceed the life-expectancy of an individual, particularly in patients aged 75 years or older. The upper age boundary for surveillance cessation is usually 75 years of age. A positive family history for an adenoma, unless a dominant genetic disease is suspected, does not require any special precautions during surveillance colonoscopies (Atkin et al., 2010).

5.3 Stratification of risk factors in patients

According to European guidelines for the quality assurance in colorectal cancer screening and diagnosis (2010), the degree of risk should be determined based on the findings at baseline colonoscopy. It is recommended to divide patients into groups with low, intermediate and high risk of colorectal neoplasia development, thus more easily determining the interval of colonoscopy examinations. Based on these results, further surveillance can be modified (Atkin et al., 2010).

Low risk group: Patients with one or two polyps measuring up to 10 mm, with tubular structure and low grade dysplasia are considered to be in low risk of developing colorectal carcinoma and may further continue in the population screening programme. However, it is necessary to also consider their age, family history, degree of bowel preparation and the quality of colonoscopy examinations.

Intermediate risk group: Patients with three or four small polyps, or one adenomatous polyp measuring ≥ 10 mm and < 20 mm, or a polyp with villous structure or high grade dysplasia, are considered to be in an intermediate risk group and should have a follow up colonoscopy in a three year interval. If there is a negative finding during the first surveillance colonoscopy another examination is indicated 5 years after the previous one. After two surveillance colonoscopies with a physiological finding, the patient can transfer to the common population colorectal cancer screening programme. If low or intermediate risk adenomas are detected, the patient should further be placed in an intermediate risk group (next surveillance colonoscopy being in a 3 year interval), in high risk polyps the next colonoscopy is recommended within 1 year.
High risk group: Patients with five small polyps or one polyp measuring at least 20mm or more are indicated to have a surveillance colonoscopy within one year from their baseline colonoscopy. If there is a negative finding or an adenoma with intermediate risk is detected, the next examination is recommended after three years. Two negative controls shift the interval for another colonoscopy by further 5 years. When a high risk adenoma is detected during a surveillance colonoscopy, an early examination is necessary - within 1 year. The aim of an early surveillance examination is to detect concurrent lesions that were not picked up during a baseline colonoscopy.

5.4 Recommendations for surveillance in chosen colonoscopy findings

Endoscopically removed pT1 carcinoma is considered a high risk lesion based on its biological characteristics, the first surveillance colonoscopy interval thus being within 12 months from the first one (Chu et al., 2003; Di Gregorio et al., 2005; Rex et al., 2006).
For surveillance purposes, serrated adenomas (i.e., traditional serrated adenomas and mixed polyps with at least one adenomatous component) should be dealt with using standard recommendations like any other adenoma. Currently, there is no data available that would explicitly certify the need for any other surveillance programme.
There has been no proof that a small hyperplastic polyp has an increased risk of colorectal carcinoma, patients with this finding are therefore placed in standard population screening programme. Individuals with one or more hyperplastic polyps measuring more than 10mm, or with non-neoplastic serrated lesions of the colon, or with multiple small lesions in the right colon, are considered to have a higher risk of developing colorectal neoplasia. However, accurate recommendations cannot be reliably determined for the current lack of data (Atkin et al., 2010).
Large sessile lesion removed by a piece-meal resection should be checked within 2-3 months, so that small areas of residual tissue can be treated endoscopically early enough. Within the next 3 months they can easily be identified using India ink tattooing and ideally completely eradicated. When a large residual finding is detected during a follow up examination, further endoscopic or surgical treatment should be considered.

5.5 Stopping surveillance

Stopping surveillance depends on several factors, not only on the characteristics of detected polyps, but also on age, comorbidities and personal wishes. The upper age boundary for surveillance colonoscopy is considered to be 75 years or older (Atkin et al., 2010). At this stage, patients can discontinue the surveillance programme and return to the population screening programme. On the other hand, patients undergoing the surveillance programme being followed up endoscopically are not indicated to continue with the FOBT.

6. Conclusion

Colonoscopy plays a major role in colorectal cancer screening. Recently published Europeans guidelines showed that although no randomized control study on the efficacy of colonoscopy has been completed yet, the recent case-control studies found a significant reduction of 31% CRC mortality. Very promising is the NordICC trial which could confirm these results. To reduce the appearance of interval cancer, colonoscopy quality control and adequate bowel preparation is necessary. Colonoscopy can be considered an effective and safe procedure.

A well organized surveillance programme for patients with adenoma, advanced adenoma or carcinoma is just as important as a baseline colonoscopy examination with its quality and precision being the determining factors of the follow up intervals. Patients should be divided into three categories using simple criteria, depending on the presumed risk of developing colorectal cancer, while being endoscopically followed up at given intervals. It is always necessary to take into consideration age, comorbidities, personal and family history, and the personal wish of each individual.

7. Acknowledgment

Authors would like to thank Dr. Gabriela Veprekova for important contribution and literature research together with the preparation of the manuscript, and also to assoc. prof. Ladislav Dusek, MSc., PhD, dr. Jan Muzik, MSc., PhD and dr. Jakub Gregor, PhD for providing the epidemiology figures.

8. References

Alberts, D.S.; Martinez, M.E.; Roe, D.J.; Guillen-Rodriguez, J.M.; Marshall, J.R.; van Leeuwen, J.B.; Reid, M.E.; Ritenbaugh, C.; Vargas, P.A.; Bhattacharyya, A.B.; Earnest, D.L. & Sampliner, R.E. (2000). Lack of effect of a high-fiber cereal supplement on the recurrence of colorectal adenomas. Phoenix Colon Cancer Prevention Physicians' Network. *N.Engl.J.Med.*, vol. 342, no. 16, pp. 1156-1162

Arber, N.; Eagle, C.J.; Spicak, J.; Racz, I;, Dite, P.; Hajer, J.; Zavoral, M.; Lechuga, M.J.; Gerletti, P.; Tang, J.; Rosenstein, R.B.; Macdonald, K.; Bhadra, P.; Fowler, R.; Wittes, J.; Zauber, A.G.; Solomon, S.D. & Levin, B. (2006). Celecoxib for the prevention of colorectal adenomatous polyps. *N.Engl.J.Med.*, vol. 355, no. 9, pp. 885-895

Atkin, W.; Valori, R.; Kuipers, E.J.; Hoff, G.; Senore, C.; Segnan N.; Jover, R.; Schmiegel, W.; Lambert, R. & Pox, C. (2010). Colonoscopic surveillance following adenoma removal. In: Segnan N, Patnick J, von Karsa L. *European guidelines for quality assurance in colorectal cancer screening and diagnosis*, 1st ed., European Union, 2010:274-297, ISBN 978-92-79-16435-4, doi: 10.2772/1458

Atkin, W.S.; Edwards, R.; Kralj-Hans, I.; Wooldrage, K.; Hart, A.R.; Northover, J.M.; Parkin, D.M.; Wardle, J.; Duffy, S.W. & Cuzick, J. (2010). Once-only flexible sigmoidoscopy screening in prevention of colorectal cancer: a multicentre randomised controlled trial. *Lancet*, vol. 375, no. 9726, pp. 1624-1633

Baron, J.A.; Sandler, R.S.; Bresalier, R.S.; Quan, H.; Riddell, R.; Lanas, A.; Bolognese, J.A.; Oxenius, B.; Horgan, K.; Loftus, S. & Morton, D.G. (2006). A randomized trial of rofecoxib for the chemoprevention of colorectal adenomas. *Gastroenterology*, vol. 131, no. 6, pp. 1674-1682

Baxter, N.N.; Goldwasser, M.A.; Paszat, L.F.; Saskin, R.; Urbach, D.R. & Rabeneck, L. (2009). Association of colonoscopy and death from colorectal cancer. *Ann.Intern.Med.*, vol. 150, no. 1, pp. 1-8

Brenner, H.; Hoffmeister, M; Arndt, V.; Stegmaier, C.; Altenhofen, L. & Haug, U. (2010). Protection from right- and leftsided colorectal neoplasms after colonoscopy: population-based study. *J.Natl.Cancer Inst.*, vol. 102, no. 2, pp. 89-95

Brenner, H.; Chang-Claude, J.; Seiler, C.M.; Sturmer, T. & Hoffmeister, M. (2006). Does a negative screening colonoscopy ever need to be repeated? *Gut*, vol. 55, no. 8, pp. 1145-1150

Cafferty, F.H.; Wong, J.M.; Yen, A.M.; Duffy, S.W.; Atkin, W.S. & Chen, T.H. (2007). Findings at follow-up endoscopies in subjects with suspected colorectal abnormalities: effects of baseline findings and time to follow-up. *Cancer J*, vol. 13, no. 4, pp. 263-270

Castells, A. & Quintero, E. (2011). Colorectal Cancer Screening in Average-Risk Population: A Multicenter, Randomized Controlled Trial Comparing Immunochemical Fecal Occult Blood Testing versus Colonoscopy. WEO/OMED Colorectal Cancer Screening Committee Meeting. Available at http://www.worldendo.org/assets/downloads/pdf/resources/ccsc/2011/weo_crc11_3_2_5_castells.pdf. Last accessed June, 4, 2011

Chu, D.Z.; Chansky, K.; Alberts, D.S.; Meyskens, F.L. Jr.; Fenoglio-Preiser, C.M.; Rivkin, S.E.; Mills, G.M.; Giguere, J.K.; Goodman, G.E.; Abbruzzese, J.L. & Lippman, S.M. (2003). Adenoma recurrences after resection of colorectal carcinoma: results from the Southwest Oncology Group 9041 calcium chemoprevention pilot study. *Ann.Surg.Oncol*, vol. 10, no. 8, pp. 870-875

Curado, M.P.; Edwards, B.; Shin, H.R.; Storm,.H.; Ferlay, J.; Heanue, M. & Boyle, P. (2007). Cancer Incidence in Five Continents, Vol. IX. IARC Scientific Publications No. 160, Lyon, IARC. Available at http://www-dep.iarc.fr/, section CI5 IX. Last accessed June, 4, 2011

Di Gregorio, C.; Benatti, P.; Losi, L.; Roncucci, L.; Rossi, G.; Ponti, G.; Marino, M.; Pedroni, M.; Scarselli, A.; Roncari, B. & Ponz, L.M. (2005). Incidence and survival of patients with Dukes' A (stages T1 and T2) colorectal carcinoma: a 15-year population-based study. *Int J Colorectal Dis*, vol. 20, no. 2, pp. 147-154

Dominitz, J.A. & Robertson, D.J. (2011). Colonoscopy Versus Fecal Immunochemical Testing in Reducing Mortality From Colorectal Cancer (CONFIRM). Available at http://clinicaltrials.gov/ct2/show/NCT01239082. Last accessed June, 4, 2011

Ferlay, J.; Bray, F. & Pisani, P. GLOBOCAN 2002. Cancer incidence, mortality and prevalence worldwide. IARC Cancer Base No. 5 version 2.0. IARC press, Lyon

2004. Available at http://www-dep.iarc.fr/, section GLOBOCAN 2002 Last accessed June, 4, 2011

Ferlay, J.; Autier, P.; Boniol, M.; Heanue, M.; Colombet, M. & Boyle, P. (2007) Estimates of the cancer incidence and mortality in Europe in 2006. *Ann Oncol.* Mar;18(3):581-92. Epub 2007 Feb 7. PMID: 17287242

Karsa, L. v.; Anttila, A.; Ronco, G.; Ponti, A.; Malila, N.; Arbyn, M.; Segnan, N.; Castillo-Beltran; M., Boniol; M., Ferlay, J.; Hery, C.; Sauvaget, C.; Voti, L. & Autier, P. (2008). Cancer screening in the European Union. Report on the implementation of the Council Recommendation on cancer screening - First Report. ISBN 978-92-79-08934-3. European Communities (publ.) Printed in Luxembourg by the services of the European Commission, 2008. Available at http://ec.europa.eu/health/ph_determinants/genetics/documents/cancer_screening.pdf. Last accessed June, 4, 2011

Laiyemo, A.O.; Pinsky, P.F.; Marcus, P.M.; Lanza, E.; Cross, A.J.; Schatzkin, A. & Schoen R.E. (2009). Utilization and yield of surveillance colonoscopy in the continued follow-up study of the polyp prevention trial. *Clin.Gastroenterol.Hepatol.*, vol. 7, no. 5, pp. 562-567

Lieberman, D.A.; Weiss, D.G.; Bond, J.H.; Ahnen, D.J.; Garewal, H. & Chejfec, G. (2000). Use of colonoscopy to screen asymptomatic adults for colorectal cancer. Veterans Affairs Cooperative Study Group 380. *N.Engl.J.Med.*, vol. 343, no. 3, pp. 162-168

Matsuda, T. Japan Polyp Study: Post-polypectomy RCT- Update. (2011). WEO/OMED Colorectal Cancer Screening Committee Meeting. Available at http://www.worldendo.org/assets/downloads/pdf/resources/ccsc/2011/weo_crc11_3_1_1_matsuda.pdf. Last accessed June, 4, 2011

Martinez, M.E.; Baron, J.A.; Lieberman, D.A.; Schatzkin, A.; Lanza, E.; Winawer, S.J.; Zauber, A.G.; Jiang, R.; Ahnen, D.J.; Bond, J.H.; Church, T.R.; Robertson, D.J.; Smith-Warner, S.A.; Jacobs, E.T.; Alberts, D.S. & Greenberg, E.R. (2009). A pooled analysis of advanced colorectal neoplasia diagnoses after colonoscopic polypectomy. *Gastroenterology*, vol. 136, no. 3, pp.832-841

NordiCC Study Protocol. Version MB 260409. Available at http://www.kreftregisteret.no/en/Research/Projects/NordICC. Last accessed June, 4, 2011

Parkin, D.M.; Whelan, S.L.; Ferlay, J. & Storm, H. (2005). Cancer Incidence in Five Continents, Vol. I to VIII. IARC CancerBase No. 7, Lyon. Available at http://www-dep.iarc.fr/, section CI5 I-VIII. Last accessed June, 4, 2011

Platell, C.F.; Philpott, G. & Olynyk JK (2002). Flexible sigmoidoscopy screening for colorectal neoplasia in average-risk people: evaluation of a five-year rescreening interval. *Med.J.Aust.*, vol. 176, no. 8, pp. 371-373

Pabby, A.; Suneja, A.; Heeren, T. & Farraye, F.A. (2005). Flexible sigmoidoscopy for colorectal cancer screening in the elderly. *Dig.Dis Sci.*, vol. 50, no. 11, pp. 2147-2152

Pox, C.; Schmiegel, W. & Classen M. (2007). Current status of screening colonoscopy in Europe and in the United States. *Endoscopy* 2007 Feb;39(2):168-73. PMID: 17327977. doi:10.1055/s-2007-966182

Regula, J.; Rupinski, M.; Kraszewska, E.; Polkowski, M.; Pachlewski, J.; Orlowska, J.; Nowacki, M.P. & Butruk, E. (2006). Colonoscopy in colorectal-cancer screening for detection of advanced neoplasia. *N. Engl J Med* 2006 Nov 2;355(18):1863-72. PMID: 17079760

Rex, D.K.; Kahi, C.J.; Levin, B.; Smith, R.A.; Bond, J.H.; Brooks, D.; Burt, R.W.; Byers, T.; Fletcher, R.H.; Hyman, N.; Johnson, D.; Kirk, L.; Lieberman, D.A.; Levin, T.R.; O'Brien, M.J.; Simmang, C.; Thorson, A.G. & Winawer, S.J. (2006). Guidelines for colonoscopy surveillance after cancer resection: a consensus update by the American Cancer Society and US Multi-Society Task Force on Colorectal Cancer. *CA Cancer J Clin*, vol. 56, no. 3, pp. 160-167

Robertson, D.J.; Greenberg, E.R.; Beach, M.; Sandler, R.S.; Ahnen, D.; Haile, R.W.; Burke, C.A.; Snover, D.C.; Bresalier, R.S.; Keown-Eyssen, G.; Mandel, J.S.; Bond, J.H.; Van Stolk, R.U.; Summers, R.W.; Rothstein, R.; Church, T.R.; Cole, B.F.; Byers, T.; Mott, L. & Baron, J.A. (2005). Colorectal cancer in patients under close colonoscopic surveillance. *Gastroenterology*, vol. 129, no. 1, pp. 34-41

Rosen, L.; Bub, D.S.; Reed, J.F., III. & Nastasee, S.A. (1993). Hemorrhage following colonoscopic polypectomy. *Dis.Colon Rectum*, vol. 36, no. 12, pp. 1126-1131

Schoen, R.E.; Pinsky, P.F.; Weissfeld, J.L.; Bresalier, R.S.; Church, T.; Prorok, P. & Gohagan, J.K. (2003). Results of repeat sigmoidoscopy 3 years after a negative examination. *JAMA*, vol. 290, no. 1, pp. 41-48

Schoenfeld, P.; Cash, B.; Flood, A.; Dobhan, R.; Eastone, J.; Coyle, W.; Kikendall, J.W.; Kim, H.M.; Weiss, D.G.; Emory, T.; Schatzkin, A. & Lieberman, D. (2005). Colonoscopic screening of average-risk women for colorectal neoplasia. *N.Engl.J.Med.*, vol. 352, no. 20, pp. 2061-2068

Segnan, N.; Senore, C.; Andreoni, B.; Azzoni, A.; Bisanti, L.; Cardelli; A., Castiglione, G.; Crosta, C.; Ederle, A.; Fantin, A.; Ferrari, A.; Fracchia, M.; Ferrero, F.; Gasperoni, S.; Recchia, S.; Risio, M.; Rubeca, T.; Saracco, G. & Zappa, M. (2007). Comparing attendance and detection rate of colonoscopy with sigmoidoscopy and FIT for colorectal cancer screening. *Gastroenterology*, vol. 132, no. 7, pp. 2304-2312

Saini, S.D.; Kim, H.M. & Schoenfeld, P. (2006). Incidence of advanced adenomas at surveillance colonoscopy in patients with a personal history of colon adenomas: a meta-analysis and systematic review. *Gastrointest.Endosc.*, vol. 64, no. 4, pp. 614-626

Singh, H.; Turner, D.; Xue, L.; Targownik, L.E. & Bernstein, C.N. (2006). Risk of developing colorectal cancer following a negative colonoscopy examination: evidence for a 10-year interval between colonoscopies. *JAMA*, vol. 295, no. 20, pp. 2366-2373

Spann, S.J.; Rozen, P.; Young, G.P. & Levin, B. (2002). Colorectal cancer: how big is the problem, why prevent it, and how might it present? In: Rozen P, Young GP, Levin B, Spann SJ. *Colorectal Cancer in Clinical Practice*. London, England: Martin Dunitz Ltd; pp: 1-18

Walsh, J.M. & Terdiman, J.P. (2003). Colorectal cancer screening: scientific review. *JAMA*, vol. 289, no. 10, pp. 1288-1296

World Health Organization (2006), mortality database, United Nations, World Population Prospects. Available at http://www.un.org/esa/population/unpop.htm. Last accessed June, 4, 2011

Zavoral, M.; Suchanek, S.; Zavada, F.; Dusek, L.; Muzik, J.; Seifert & B.; Fric, P. (2009). Colorectal cancer screening in Europe. *World Journal Of Gastroenterology*, Vol.15,No.47, (December 2009), pp. 5907-5915, ISSN 1007-9327

2

Preparing for Colonoscopy

Parakkal Deepak, Humberto Sifuentes,
Muhammed Sherid and Eli D.Ehrenpreis
NorthShore University Health System
Evanston, Illinois
USA

1. Introduction

Colorectal cancer screening for average risk individuals beginning at the age of fifty has been recommended by the American Cancer Society, the American College of Gastroenterology, the American Society for Gastrointestinal Endoscopy, the American Gastroenterological Association and the American College of Radiology (Levin et al., 2008). Colorectal cancer screening has been shown to reduce the incidence and mortality of cancer of the colon and rectum due to early detection and removal of precancerous lesions and adenomas. Colonoscopy is generally considered to be the preferred method of screening despite the emergence of computed tomographic (CT) colonography and the use of other recommended screening modalities (Rex et al., 2009). Other indications for colonoscopy (ASGE, 2000) include evaluation and treatment of gastrointestinal bleeding, unexplained iron deficiency anemia, clinically significant chronic diarrhea of unexplained origin, foreign body removal, decompression of acute nontoxic megacolon or sigmoid volvulus, balloon dilation of stenotic lesions and in palliative procedures for colonic obstructive or bleeding neoplasms.

Colonoscopy requires thorough cleansing of the large intestine for full visualization as well as the safe and effective completion of the procedure. This chapter describes the rationale for bowel preparation, the types of preparations currently available, complications associated with bowel preparations and special considerations for bowel preparation in specific segments of the population. The consequences of inadequate bowel preparation, use of antibiotic prophylaxis for the procedure and management of anticoagulants and antiplatelet agents before and after colonoscopy will also be reviewed. Literature was accessed using MEDLINE (through March, 2011) for all relevant articles published in the English language.

2. Preparing for colonoscopy

2.1 Why prepare?

Inadequate bowel preparation is responsible for up to one third of all incomplete colonoscopy procedures (Belsey et al., 2007). Poor preparation precludes up to 10% of examinations (Kazarian et al., 2008), negatively impacts the rate of overall polyp (Froehlich et al., 2005; Harewood et al., 2003) and adenomatous polyp detection (Thomas-Gibson et al., 2006). In additional, poor bowel preparation raises costs due to aborted examinations followed by repeated procedures. In a study of 200 consecutive outpatient colonoscopies, imperfect bowel preparation resulted in a 12% increase in costs at a university hospital and 22% increase in costs at a public hospital (Rex et al., 2002).

2.2 Types of bowel preparations

The ideal colon preparation should rapidly and reliably cleanse the colon of fecal material while having no effect on the gross or microscopic appearance of the colon (Wexner et al., 2006). It should require a short period for ingestion and evacuation, cause no discomfort, and produce no significant fluid or electrolyte shifts while also being palatable, simple, and inexpensive.

Agents used for bowel preparation can be divided into three main categories according to their mechanism of action, these being isosmotic, hyperosmotic, and adjunctive preparations. Polyethylene glycol-electrolyte lavage solutions (PEG-ELSs) and sodium phosphate (NaP) formulations are among the most commonly used.

2.2.1 Isosmotic bowel preparations

Isosmotic preparations that contain polyethylene glycol (PEG) are osmotically balanced, high-volume, nonfermentable electrolyte solutions **(Table 1).** These preparations cleanse the bowel with minimal water and electrolyte absorption or secretion in the bowel lumen and provide evacuation, primarily by the mechanical effects of a large-volume lavage. Standard dosing of the 4 liter PEG-ELS is 240 ml(8 oz.) every 10 minutes or a rate of 20 to 30 mL/min if administered by nasogastric tube. This intake rate is generally continued until the rectal output is clear or the entire volume of the preparation is ingested (Wexner et al., 2006). Because of the salty taste of PEG-ELS, sulfate-free PEG preparations were developed; patients by a 3:1 ratio preferred the sulfate free 4 liter PEG-ELS compared to the original formulation (76% versus 24%, $p \leq 0.0001$) with no difference in the efficacy of colonic cleansing (Di Palma and Marshall, 1990). To improve taste, flavored preparations have also been introduced. Unfortunately, flavorings may increase the osmotic load, and some contain carbohydrates that, with bacterial fermentation, could lead to production of combustible gases (Wexner, 1996).

A further development for the advancement PEG-ELSs came with reduced volume preparations. Good or excellent cleansing was reported in 87% of the patients receiving 2-liter PEG-ELSs combined with bisacodyl (irritant laxative tablets) (n=93) compared to 92% of patients receiving a 4-liter sulfate free PEG-ELSs ($p=0.16$). The lower volume preparation was associated with decreased abdominal fullness ($p < 0.01$), nausea ($p < 0.01$), vomiting ($p = 0.01$), and overall discomfort ($p < 0.01$) (Di Palma et al., 2003). For this regimen, dosing on the evening prior to the procedure consists of two 5 mg bisacodyl delayed release tablets followed after the first bowel movement by 240 mL of PEG-ELS preparation every 10 minutes until the excreted effluent is clear or until a total of 2 L is ingested. Only clear liquids are permitted on the day of the preparation. Another low volume PEG-ELS consists of the addition of ascorbic acid in the 2-L PEG solution, that is also dosed 240 mL every 10 minutes split into two one 1 liter doses, each accompanied by 16 oz. of clear fluid for hydration.. This regimen permits a normal breakfast and lunch followed by a light dinner (clear soup or yogurt or both) on the day prior to the procedure, followed by bowel prep starting 1 hour after the evening meal. The second liter dose can be consumed 1.5 hours after the initial 1 liter or on the morning of the colonoscopy (Wexner et al., 2006).The 2 liter PEG with ascorbic acid was compared to 4-liter PEG-ELS in a trial where successful gut cleansing was achieved in 136 of 153 (88.9%) cases of the 2 liter PEG with ascorbic acid group and 147 of 155 (94.8%) cases of the 4 L PEG-ELS group. The 2 liter regimen was also associated with lower frequency of nausea (14% versus 23%; 95% confidence interval [CI], -17 to -1) and abdominal pain (3% versus 8%; 95% CI, -10 to -0.2).Patient ratings of acceptability and taste were better for the 2-liter PEG with ascorbic acid group than for the PEG-ELS group ($P < 0.025$) with a higher completion rate of entire preparation ($p=0.035$) (Ell et al, 2008). Collectively, these studies suggest that the 2 liter preparations of PEG-ELS are as effective as and better tolerated than the 4 liter PEG-ELS preparations.

Efficacy of the standard 4-L PEG-ELS preparation can be improved by administration of split doses, even with minimal dietary restriction before the first dose (El Sayed et al., 2003). Ingestion of the entire preparation on the day of the procedure about 5 hours before the colonoscopy has also been shown to improve the clean-out quality when compared with patients who received PEG-ELS the previous day (approximately19 hours before the procedure) (Church, 1998).

2.2.2 Hyperosmotic bowel preparations

Hyperosmotic bowel preparations have a mechanism of action of drawing water and electrolytes into the bowel lumen, stimulating fluid loss, peristalsis and evacuation. These small-volume preparations cause fluid shifts, accompanied by electrolyte alterations (Ehrenpreis et al., 1998; Lichtenstein, 2009). Of these, the most commonly used include oral NaP available in as tablets and an aqueous solution (now withdrawn from the US market). The aqueous NaP preparation contains monobasic and dibasic NaP. The solution form of NaP contains 90 ml of solution with each 45-mL dose containing contains 29.7 g NaP. Two doses of 45 mL aqueous solution are given at least 10 to 12 hours apart, with the second dose given within 5 hours of the procedure. Each of these solutions should be diluted in 8 oz of clear liquid with a minimum of l 16 oz of clear liquids to be consumed after each dose (Wexner et al., 2006). The first study(Vanner et al., 1990) compared the 4 L PEG-ELS with the 90 ml NaP solution included 102 patients randomized to receive either oral NaP solution($n=54$) or standard PEG-ELSs ($n=48$) prior to colonoscopy. Overall, good to excellent bowel cleansing was reported in a significantly higher number of patients who received sodium phosphate(80%) compared to the patients who received PEG-ELS(33%), ($p<0.001$). Completion of bowel preparation was also significantly higher in the NaP group (85%) compared to the PEG-ELS group (31%), ($p<0.001$). A recent meta-analysis reviewed randomized controlled clinical trials from 1990 to 2005 and compared the tolerability, efficacy, and safety of various preparations. Pooled data from 15 trials with 3293 patients that compared PEG and NaP preparations showed that 94.4% of patients completed taking NaP compared with 70.9% of patients taking PEG solution Using a random effects model, the odds ratio of completion of preparation was 0.16 (95% CI: 0.09–0.29; $P < 0.00001$) in favor of NaP (Tan and Tjandra, 2006).

Two NaP tablet preparations are FDA approved for cleansing prior to colonoscopy. The original formulation (Visicol™) contained microcrystalline cellulose (MCC), an excipient and was thought to reduce mucosal visibility during colonoscopy, with a new MCC-free preparation now available (Osmoprep™). The dose is 40 tablets (60 g) for the MCC containing preparation and 32 tablets (48 g) for the MCC-free preparation, both divided into 2 doses separated by 10 to 12 hours. 20 tablets are taken the night before the colonoscopy, 4

tablets every 15 minutes followed by 8 oz clear liquids and the remaining 12-20 tablets on the morning of the colonoscopy within 3-5 hours of the procedure. A split-dose NaP schedule, with one dose taken the day before and one on the day of the procedure separated by 12 hours, was also found to be superior relative to a single dose (Frommer, 1997). All NaP regimens should be taken with a minimum of 2 L of clear liquids. In the event that the bowel preparation is inadequate after the full dose of the NaP formulation, the reparation should be completed using a non-NaP formulation such as PEG-ELS (Wexner et al., 2006)
Clinical studies have shown the original MCC containing NaP tablet formulation to be as efficacious and better tolerated than 4 liter PEG-ELS formulation and be equally as effective as an aqueous NaP solution. (Aronchick et al., 2000). The 32 tablet MCC free NaP tablet formulation has been shown to be at least as efficacious and better tolerated than the MCC containing formulation (Wruble et al., 2007) and also with better colon cleansing and tolerability compared to the 2 liter PEG-ELS formulation (Johanson JF et al.,2007). A prospective trial (Rex et al., 2006(B)) reported that patients receiving the 32 tablet NaP formulation (n=239) compared with the 40 tablet formulation (n=236) had significantly smaller increase in serum phosphate levels from baseline (3.5 mg/dl versus 4.4 mg/dl, $p \leq 0.0002$). This improvement must be tempered by the common occurrence of electrolyte and fluid imbalances as well as serious side effects from NaP containing preparations (see below).

Recently a new sulfate based osmotic laxative(SUPREP) was approved by the FDA in August, 2010 for bowel preparation before colonoscopy containing sodium sulfate 17.5 g, potassium sulfate 3.13 g, magnesium sulfate 1.6 g in each 6 oz bottle. Sodium absorption in the small intestine with sodium sulfate preparations is largely reduced because of the absence of chloride, the accompanying anion necessary for active absorption against electrochemical gradient. Unlike oral sodium phosphate, sulfate salts do not produce renal tubular injury in animal models (Pelham, et al, 2009).

A split dose (2-Day) regimen is advocated. The efficacy of the oral sulfate solution (OSS) was compared with 4 liter sulfate free PEG-ELS in a multicenter, single-blind, randomized, non-inferiority study involving one hundred thirty-six outpatients undergoing colonoscopy. Successful or excellent bowel preparation was more frequent with OSS than with sulfate free PEG-ELS (98.4% versus 89.6%; $P = .04$ and 71.4% versus 34.3%; $P < .001$ respectively). Gastrointestinal side effects and adverse events were not significantly different between the 2 groups (Rex et al., 2010).

Other hyperosmolar bowel preparations include sodium picosulfate, a salt that has similar action as NaP, producing a cathartic effect by osmotic effect in the bowel. This preparation is commonly used alone and in combination with magnesium citrate outside of the United States, especially in the United Kingdom for bowel preparation for colonoscopy. A pooled analysis of 381 patients receiving sodium picosulfate and 369 patients receiving sodium phosphate demonstrated a significantly higher efficacy in bowel cleansing (described as good or excellent cleansing), with the NaP formulation (90%) compared with sodium picosulfate (82%) ($p = 0.004$). A similar adverse event profile was seen with the two preparations (Tan and Tjandra, 2006). The pooled analysis also demonstrated a similar efficacy of sodium picosulfate when compared to 4 liter PEG-ELSs with an additional reduction in the number of adverse events (48% versus 71% respectively, $p = 0.003$).

Product (manufacturer)	Active agent	FDA approved (adults)	Quantity
Isosmotic			
Full volume			
Colyte (Scwarz Pharm, Mequon, Wis)	PEG-3350	Yes	
Flavored			4000 ml
Nonflavored			4000 ml
GoLYTELY (Braintree, Braintree, Mass)	PEG-3350	Yes	
Flavored			4000 ml
Unflavored			4000 ml
NuLYTELY (Braintree)	PEG-3350(sulfate free)	Yes	
Flavored			4000 ml
Nonflavored			4000 ml
TriLyte (Scwarz Pharm)	PEG-3350(sulfate free)	Yes	
Flavored			4000 ml
Low volume			
Halflytely (Braintree)	PEG-3350 and bisacodyl	Yes	2000 ml
MoviPrep (Salix , Morrisville, NC)	PEG-3350 and ascorbic acid	Yes	2000 ml
Hyperosmotic			
Fleet Phospho-Soda EZ-Prep(oral)	NaP 29.7 grams/45 ml	‡	75 ml§
Visicol (tablet, NaP; Salix)	NaP (oral) 1.5 grams/tablet	Yes	40 tablets
Osmoprep (MCC-free tablet, NaP; Salix)	NaP (oral) 1.5 grams/tablet	Yes	32 tablets
Fleet enema (C.B. Fleet)	Monobasic NaP Monohydrate-19 g Dibasic NaP Heptahydrate-7 g	Yes	118 ml
SUPREP kit(Braintree, Braintree, Mass)	In 6 oz-Na sulfate-17.5g, K sulfate-3.13 g, Mg sulfate 1.6 g	Yes	360 ml

LoSoPrep kit (E-Z-EM Inc, Lake Success, NY)	Mg citrate -18 g plus 20 mg bisacodyl oral and 10 mg suppository	Yes	38.5 ml
Magnesium citrate	Mg citrate-17.45 g	Yes	300 ml
Adjunctive medications			
Senna (AmerisourceBergen, Chesterbrook,PA)	Sennosides 8.6 mg	Yes	Tablets
Bisacodyl (Amkas)	Bisacodyl 5 mg	Yes	Tablets

‡ FDA recommends against use of over-the-counter oral NaP for bowel preparation.
§ C.B. Fleet ceased distribution and initiated a recall on December 11, 2008.

Table 1. Agents used for bowel preparation

Magnesium citrate is another hyperosmotic agent that also promotes release of cholecystokinin, resulting in fluid and electrolyte secretion as well as stimulation of peristalsis. It is typically not effective as a sole agent for colonic cleansing; hence it is used mainly in combination with other agents. Magnesium is renally excreted and should be used in extreme caution in patients with renal insufficiency or renal failure.. Sodium picosulfate in combination with magnesium citrate has been compared to 2 liter PEG-ELS with ascorbic acid with similar efficacy (73 % versus 84% respectively, p=0.367) and adverse event profile. Improved preparation was seen in the ascending colon (p=0.024) and cecum (p=0.003) (Worthington et al., 2008). Magnesium citrate in combination with 2 liter PEG-ELS solution has also been shown to improve preparation quality and improve patient satisfaction compared to 4 liter PEG-ELSs (Sharma et al., 1998). Combination preparations containing magnesium citrate also include a 240-mL dose of balanced magnesium solution and 20 mg bisacodyl(oral) the evening before the procedure and a 10-mg bisacodyl suppository the morning of the procedure (Delegge and Kaplan, 2005).A pulsed rectal irrigation with magnesium citrate as also been suggested to enhance preparation for colonoscopy; however, this requires skilled nursing for administration and is associated with a high cost (Chang et al, 1991).

2.3 Additional medications/methods used in bowel cleansing

2.3.1 Bisacodyl

Bisacodyl is a poorly absorbed diphenylmethane which acts locally on the colon as a peristaltic stimulant. Its active metabolites stimulate colonic motility with an onset of action between 6 and 10 hours. It is often used as an adjunct with PEG-ELS although this combination has not demonstrated a significant difference in the quality of the preparation or amount of residual colonic fluid during colonoscopy (Ziegenhagen et al., 1992).Use of bisacodyl as an adjunct to PEG-ELS may allow patients to consume a smaller volume of PEG necessary for colonic cleansing (Sharma et al., 1998).

2.3.2 Senna

Senna is an anthraquinone derivative that is activated by colonic bacteria. These activated derivates have a direct effect on intestinal mucosa increasing the rate of colonic motility, enhancing colonic transit and inhibiting water and electrolyte secretion. Like bisacodyl, senna can also be used as an adjunct to PEG-ELS. It has also been shown to reduce the amount of PEG-ELS required for effective bowel preparation (Iida et al., 1992).

2.3.3 Flavoring

Several methods to improve the palatability of both PEG-ELS and NaP solutions have been attempted. PEG-ELSs are now available in multiple flavors including cherry, citrus-berry, lemon-lime, orange and pineapple. Carbohydrate-electrolyte solutions such as Gatorade® and Crystal Light® have also been recommended to improve the taste in PEG and NaP solutions(Wexner et al.,2006).Other methods to improve taste that are often used in clinical practice include slowing the rate of consumption, chilling the solution and consuming lemon slices with preparations.

2.4 Assessment of bowel preparation quality

The American Society for Gastrointestinal Endoscopy (ASGE) and American College of Gastroenterology (ACG) Taskforce on Quality in Endoscopy have suggested that every colonoscopy report should include an assessment of the quality of bowel preparation. They proposed the use of terms such as "excellent," "good," "fair," and "poor," but admitted that these terms lack standardized definitions (Rex et al., 2006(A)).

One validated measurement of preparation quality is the Boston Bowel Preparation Scale (BBPS), which was developed to limit inter-observer variability in the rating of bowel preparation quality, while preserving the ability to distinguish various degrees of bowel cleanliness (Lai et al., 2009). The subjective terms previously described were replaced by a 3 point scoring system applied to each of the 3 regions of the colon: the right colon (including the cecum and ascending colon), the transverse colon (including the hepatic and splenic flexures), and the left colon (including the descending colon, sigmoid colon, and rectum). The points are defined as follows: 0 = unprepared colon segment with mucosa not seen because of solid stool that cannot be cleared; 1 = portion of mucosa of the colon segment seen, but other areas of the colon segment not well seen because of staining, residual stool, and/or opaque liquid; 2 = minor amount of residual staining, small fragments of stool and/or opaque liquid, but mucosa of colon segment seen well; 3 = entire mucosa of colon segment seen well with no residual staining, small fragments of stool or opaque liquid. Each of the 3 segment scores is then summed for a total score of 0 to 9, in which 0 is unprepared and 9 is entirely clean. If an endoscopist aborts a procedure due to an inadequate preparation, then any nonvisualized proximal segments are assigned a score of 0. An instructional video demonstrating the BPPS is available and can be accessed online at http://bmc.org/gastroenterology/research.htm (Lai et al., 2009). In a comprehensive validation study, the BBPS was found to be a reliable instrument for assessing bowel cleanliness during colonoscopy (Calderwood & Jacobson, 2010).

2.5 Complications of bowel preparation

2.5.1 Inadequate bowel preparation

An inadequate preparation for colonoscopy can result in many complications including missed lesions, cancelled procedures, increased procedure time, and an increased potential in complication rates. Currently, there are no specific guidelines for the management of patients in whom an adequate examination of the colon cannot be achieved due to an inadequate preparation. The ASGE has recommended the following "reasonable" approach: the same preparation can be repeated if the patient did not consume the preparation as prescribed, except not within 24 hours when using NaP because risk of toxicity. In patients who properly consumed the preparation, options include repeating the preparation with a longer interval of consuming clear liquids only before the preparation, switching to an alternative but equally effective preparation, adding another cathartic such as magnesium citrate, bisacodyl or senna to the previous regimen, or double administration of the preparation during a two-day period (with the exception of NaP). Combining preparations (example, PEG ELS and NaP solutions) may also be successful.

2.5.2 Toxicities of bowel preparation

With the exception of NaP containing preparations, most bowel preparations have been demonstrated to be safe to use in healthy individuals without significant comorbid conditions. Caution must always be taken in selecting a bowel preparation for patients with renal, hepatic or cardiac disease and those patients at the extremes of age. New data also suggests female gender and smaller body size are risk factors for complications of NaP preparations (Parakkal & Ehrenpreis, 2010).

2.5.2.1 Oral sodium phosphate

As of December 11, 2008 the FDA issued an alert about the safe use of oral NaP products and added a black box warning for acute phosphate nephropathy (Food and Drug Administration, 2008). The FDA alert also highlighted several patients at risk of developing this complication including individuals over the age of 55; patients who are hypovolemic or have decreased intravascular volume; people who have baseline kidney disease, bowel obstruction or active colitis; and those that are using medications that affect renal perfusion (such as diuretics, angiotensin converting enzyme [ACE] inhibitors, angiotensin receptor blockers [ARBs], and possibly nonsteroidal anti-inflammatory drugs [NSAIDs]). Females of smaller body size are an additional risk group (Ehrenpreis, 2009).

Oral NaP preparations can cause fluid and electrolyte shifts secondary to the hyperosmotic nature of the products. It is often associated with the following abnormalities: hypernatremia, hypokalemia, hypocalcemia, decreased serum bicarbonate, and hyperphosphatemia (Ehrenpreis et al., 1997). Although electrolyte shifts are typically transient, clinically significant toxicities have been reported (Vanner et al., 1990). NaP preparations can also cause colonic mucosal abnormalities such as aphthoid erosions similar to those seen in inflammatory bowel disease and histologic findings including focal active inflammation, mucosal disruption and erosion, edema of the lamia propria, mucosal hyperemia, focal hemorrhage, lymphoid nodules and ulceration (Rejchrt et al., 2004). Physicians are advised to avoid using NaP preparations when evaluating patients with inflammatory bowel disease or patients with diarrhea of unknown etiology.

2.5.2.2 PEG

The most common adverse effects with PEG ELS are abdominal fullness, nausea and bloating. Rare events include Mallory-Weiss tears, esophageal perforation, toxic colitis, pill malabsorption, pulmonary aspiration, hypothermia, cardiac arrhythmias, PEG-induced pancreatitis and inappropriate antidiuretic hormone secretion (Clark & DiPalma, 2004). The use of PEG-based solutions is contraindicated in patients with gastric outlet obstructions, small and large intestinal obstruction, and suspected bowel perforation.

2.5.2.3 Magnesium Preparations

Magnesium citrate should be used with caution in patients with renal insufficiency or renal failure because it is eliminated by the kidney. Fatal reports and episodes of hypermagnesemia have been reported in patients with suspected or known renal failure or elderly patients (Schelling, 2000).

3. Other considerations

3.1 Antibiotic prophylaxis

Transient bacteremia can occur during colonoscopy due to bacterial translocation of normal colonic flora into the bloodstream. Translocated bacteria may potentially adhere in remote tissues such as the endocardium. Antibiotic prophylaxis was commonly used in some high risk patients before colonoscopy, primarily to prevent infective endocarditis. However, the American Heart Association (AHA) and the American Society of Gastrointestinal Endoscopy (ASGE), in 2007 and 2008 respectively, have revised their recommendations regarding antibiotic prophylaxis before procedures including colonoscopy (Banerjee et al, 2008; Wilson et al, 2007). Both societies classify cardiac patients as low, moderate, or high risk for endocarditis. New guidelines suggest that, antibiotic prophylaxis before including colonoscopy with or without biopsies or polypectomy is no longer recommended in any risk group including those considered to be high-risk. This change in practice came about mainly because of a lack of convincing evidence to demonstrate a risk of endocarditis from gastrointestinal procedures. In addition, harmless bacteremia occurs in some daily activities such as tooth brushing. For example, in a study done by Lockhart et al., routine tooth brushing was associated with bacteremia in 23% of subjects (Lockhart et al, 2008). Bhanji et al. reported a 46% bacteremia rate (Bhanji et al, 2002), and Banerjee reported a 68% rate (Banerjee et al, 2008). Bacteremia can occur after colonoscopy, with rates ranging from 0-25%, and an average mean rate of 4.4% (Banerjee et al, 2008; Nelson, 2003). In contrast, a study done by Goldman showed that blood cultures were positive in 1% of patients after sigmoidoscopy (Goldman, 1985). Microorganisms causing transient bacteremia during and after gastrointestinal procedures are generally believed to have little potential to cause infective endocarditis. Normal skin floras are the most common organisms isolated from blood cultures after colonoscopy (although these could be a contamination during blood draw), (Llach et al, 1999; Levy, 2007). Despite more than 16 million colonoscopies and sigmoidoscopies that are done in each year in the United Stated (Seeff et al, 2004), there have been only 15 cases of infective endocarditis having a temporal relation with these procedures. The potential side effects of prophylactic antibiotics to prevent an extremely small number of cases of infective endocarditis are felt to clearly outweigh their possible benefit (Banerjee et al, 2008; Wilson et al, 2007; Van der Meer, 1992).

In cirrhotic patients with or without ascites in the absence of gastrointestinal bleeding who undergo colonoscopy, the risk of bacteremia is low. Llach et al. prospectively studied 58 patients underwent colonoscopy. Four of these patients had positive blood cultures; none developed symptoms or signs of infections (Llach et al, 1999).

Patients on peritoneal dialysis may be at risk for infectious complications of colonoscopy. In fact, there are several case reports of peritonitis in patients on peritoneal dialysis after colonoscopy especially following polypectomy (Bac et al, 1994; Ray et al, 1990). The 2005 International Society for Peritoneal Dialysis (ISPD) recommendations state that these patients have antibiotic prophylaxis before any procedure involving abdomen and pelvis including colonoscopy, and emptying the peritoneal fluid prior to the procedure (Piraino et al, 2005); however, these prevention strategies were not addressed in 2010 ISPD guidelines (Li et al, 2010).

Antibiotic prophylaxis is not recommended by the ASGE before colonoscopy or any other GI procedures in patients who have prosthetic vascular grafts or cardiovascular devices such as pacemakers (Banerjee et al, 2008). However, the AHA recommends antibiotic prophylaxis for procedures occurring within the first 6 months of prosthetic vascular grafts while graft epithelialization is occurring (Wilson et al, 2007).

Antibiotic prophylaxis is not recommended for patients who have prosthetic orthopedic devices undergoing colonoscopy, due to their low risk of infection (Banerjee et al, 2008). However, scattered cases of infections in prosthetic joints after colonoscopy have been reported (Vanderhooft et al, 1994; Cornelius et al, 2003).

3.2 Management of antiplatelet agents

Antiplatelet agents are used widely to treat patients with cardiovascular and cerebrovascular diseases as well as acute and chronic pain. Aspirin and other nonsteroidal anti-inflammatory drugs (NSAID) are not believed to increase the risk of significant bleeding after colonoscopy whether biopsies and/or polypectomies are performed. Use of aspirin was not a risk factor for polypectomy-associated bleeding in a study of 1657 patients (Hui et al, 2004). Recommendations regarding the management of antithrombotic agents before endoscopic procedures published by the ASGE in 2009 classify the procedures from low-risk to higher-risk (see **Table2**). In addition, cardiovascular conditions are also classified from low-risk to higher-risk (see **Table 3**), (Anderson et al, 2009). Colonoscopy with or without biopsy is considered a low risk procedure, however if polypectomy is done, the risk is considered higher. The ASGE recommends that aspirin and NSAIDs should not be discontinued prior to colonoscopy if one of them is used alone and if their use is necessary in any of risk groups. There is some evidence that combination of aspirin and other NSAIDs increases the risk of bleeding after polypectomy (Grossman et al, 2010), thus discontinuation of NSAIDs two to three days before polypectomy is recommended in patients on combined therapy.

Dipyridamole, another antiplatelet agent, used either alone or in combination with aspirin may be continued in patients undergoing colonoscopy with no significant risk of bleeding, however its safety is unknown in high risk procedures such as polypectomy (Zuckerman et al, 2005).

Thienopyridines (Ticlopidine, clopidogrel, prasugrel) are newer antiplatelet agents. The AHA recommends their use for a minimum of one month after placement of bare metal stents and one year for drug-eluting stents (King et al, 2008). Use of clopidogrel alone is not associated with an increased risk of post-polypectomy bleeding, however when combined with other antiplatelet agents, bleeding risk is increased (Singh et al, 2010). Due to the high rate of stent thrombosis associated with early cessation of dual antiplatelet (clopidogrel with aspirin), it is recommended that discontinuation should be avoided whenever possible (Iakovou et al, 2005). The ASGE recommends not discontinuing thienopyridines in patients undergoing low-risk procedures including colonoscopy with or without biopsy (Anderson et al, 2009). In patients undergoing high-risk procedures including polypectomy, endoscopists are advised to consider the patient's risk for thromboembolic phenomenon. If the patient is considered to have a low-risk condition, thienopyridines can be discontinued 7-10 days before the procedure. Alternatively, procedures should be postponed until the time when thromboembolic risk is low (Anderson et al, 2009). In low-risk patients who discontinue thienopyridines, continuation of aspirin alone if they are on dual antiplatelet therapy or initiation of aspirin before procedure should be considered. This may decrease the risk of thromboembolic events without increasing the chance of developing significant bleeding. Thienopyridines should be restarted as soon as safely possible with consideration for their underlying indication and the procedure that has been performed (Anderson et al, 2009).

Glycoprotein IIb/IIIa receptor inhibitors (Epitifibatide, tirofiban, abciximab) are administered in some patients of acute coronary syndrome, however when elective colonoscopy is considered, patients are typically not taking one of these drugs. When patients require emergent colonoscopy for acute GI bleeding, these antiplatelet agents should be discontinued (Anderson et al, 2009).

In patients who develop GI bleeding while on any anti-platelet agents, the decision to continue, stop, or reverse the antiplatelet effect should be tailored case-by-case, based on the severity of bleeding, the risk of thromboembolic events. A discussion with relevant consultants in this setting is advised. Diagnostic and therapeutic colonoscopy in the setting of acute lower GI bleeding while using antiplatelet agents has been deemed to be safe and is recommended (Anderson et al, 2009).

Low risk procedure	**High risk procedures**
Diagnostic(EGD, colonoscopy, flexible sigmoidoscopy) including biopsy	Polypectomy
Enteroscopy and diagnostic balloon-assisted enteroscopy	Therapeutic balloon-assisted enteroscopy
ERCP without sphincterotomy	Endoscopic homeostasis
Enteral stent deployment(without dilation)	Tumor ablation by any technique
Capsule endoscopy	Pneumatic or bougie dilation
EUS without FNA	Biliary or pancreatic sphincterotomy
	PEG placement
	EUS with FNA
	Cystogastrostomy
	Treatment of varices

Table 2. Procedure risk for bleeding: adapted from ASGE guidelines (Anderson et al, 2009).

Low risk condition	High risk condition
Uncomplicated or paroxysmal non-valvular atrial fibrillation	Atrial fibrillation associated with valvular heart disease, prosthetic valves, active congestive heart failure, left ventricular ejection fraction <35%, history of a thromboembolic event, hypertension, diabetes mellitus, or age>75 year
Bio prosthetic valve	Mechanical valve in any position and previous thromboembolic event
Mechanical valve in aortic position	Mechanical valve in mitral position
Deep vein thrombosis	Recent (<1 year) placed coronary stent
	Acute coronary syndrome
	Non-stented percutaneous coronary intervention after myocardial infarction

Table 3. Condition risk for thromboembolic event: adapted from ASGE guidelines (Anderson et al, 2009).

3.3 Management of anticoagulants

The approach to the performance of colonoscopy in patients receiving anticoagulation agents (warfarin, heparin, low-molecular weight heparins) is another commonly encountered dilemma for the gastroenterologist. Using warfarin is not believed to increase the risk of significant bleeding in patients undergoing colonoscopy and other low-risk procedures (see table 2). The ASGE recommends continuation of warfarin for these procedures (Anderson et al, 2009). In high-risk procedures including polypectomy, there is an increased risk of bleeding (Hui et al, 2004). If patient is in a low thromboembolic risk group (see table 3), warfarin should be discontinued before a high-risk procedure, until the international normalized ratio (INR) is normal or nearly normal (Anderson et al, 2009). Vitamin K should be avoided since it delays the development of a therapeutic INR once warfarin is resumed. If patient is in a high thromboembolic risk group, bridging therapy (discontinue warfarin and administer heparin or LMWH) should be considered, however deferring the procedure to a time when the thromboembolic risk is low, is a better strategy whenever possible, depending on the degree of emergency of colonoscopy. The appropriate time to reinitiate warfarin and other anticoagulants after colonoscopy and other procedures is not clear. The ASGE recommends resumption of warfarin on the evening after procedure and heparin 2-6 hours after the procedure; however the risk of bleeding versus the risk of thromboembolic events should be weighed carefully and discussion with relevant consultants is suggested (Anderson et al, 2009).

4. Special considerations for colonoscopy preparations

4.1 Elderly

Age does not, by itself, increase the risk to colonoscopy. Colonoscopy can be performed in octogenarians and older patients (Lagares-Garcia et al, 2001; Lukens et al, 2002). A significant problem encountered in the performance of colonoscopy in the elderly is the achievement of adequate bowel preparation. Dementia, cerebrovascular accident, diabetes mellitus, renal failure, chronic obstructive pulmonary disease, chronic constipation, use of narcotics and tricyclic antidepressants are conditions that are associated with poor bowel preparation (Reilly & Walker, 2004; Ness et al; 2001; Taylor & Schubert, 2001). All of these conditions are more common among elderly, however, even after eliminating all these independent predictors for inadequate bowel preparation, age still remains an independent risk factor for inadequate preparation, (Qureshi et al, 2000; Ure et al, 1995).

Colonoscopy preparations often cause fecal incontinence in elderly patients, regardless of the type of bowel preparation, due to the large volume rectal output in a short time that these preparations induce. Thomson et al. found that approximately 25% of elderly experienced at least one episode of fecal incontinence during bowel preparation for colonoscopy (Thomson et al, 1996).

The elderly are at increased risk of severe electrolyte imbalances from sodium phosphate containing colonoscopy preparations (Beloosesky et al, 2003; Gumurdulu et al, 2004). Elderly are also more likely to have comorbidities including renal failure, congestive heart failure, and cirrhosis that increase risk for electrolyte abnormalities and sudden change in intravascular volume. Additionally, the elderly are more likely to be on medications such as diuretics, nonsteroidal anti-inflammatory drugs(NSAIDs) and angiotensin converting enzyme inhibitors that are other potential causes for electrolyte abnormalities and change in intravascular volume when NaP is used (Anderson et al 2009; Ainley et al, 2005; Desmeules et al, 2003). Of interest, studies have suggested that the efficacy of sodium phosphate is similar to nonelderly adults and comparable with PEG (Thomson et al, 1996; Seinela et al, 2003).

Magnesium citrate causes electrolyte and fluid disturbances, especially in patients with renal dysfunction. Cases of hypermagnesemia have been reported in elderly patients after magnesium citrate preparations even without known kidney disease (Kontani et al, 2005; Schelling, 2000).

Polyethylene glycol (PEG) does not, in general, cause fluid and electrolytes imbalance. However, a study done by Ho et al. showed that hypokalemia can occur after PEG preparation (Ho et al, 2010). Due to its large volume, PEG is contraindicated in patients with impaired swallowing function, (as seen in patients with stroke, dementia and Parkinson's disease) all of which are more common among the elderly. If colonoscopy is necessary in patients with these problems, a nasogastric tube can be inserted to administer the solution. However, it is possible that this approach does not decrease the risk of aspiration (Marschall et al, 1998).

4.2 Female patients

There is no data regarding the differences between men and women related to the success of bowel preparation for colonoscopy. However, there are data regarding differences in completion of colonoscopy, procedure tolerance, difficulty of the procedure rated by colonoscopist, and detection of polyps. Completion of colonoscopy is less likely in females, especially if there is a history of hysterectomy (Church, 1994). Women have longer colons comparing to men, resulting in requirement for more time to perform colonoscopy, more discomfort to the patients, and increased technical difficulties in performance of the procedure. In a study performed by Saunders et al., female colons were 10 cm longer than men's (P=0.005). Technically difficult examinations were reported in 31% of women comparing to 16% of men (Saunders et al, 1996). Female gender was also an independent predictor of difficult colonoscopy in a study performed by Anderson (Anderson et al 2001).

In another study, looping of the colonoscope was more frequent ($P = 0.0002$) and the procedure was more painful ($P = 0.0140$) in women than in men (Shah et al, 2002). Detection of polyps and adenomas were lower in post-hysterectomy women compared to women without a hysterectomy ($P= 0.008$). In addition, sigmoidoscopy was more painful ($p < 0.001$), more difficult ($p < 0.001$), and less extensive ($p < 0.0001$) in this group, (Adams et al, 2003). Women, especially of smaller stature are at increased risk of electrolyte abnormalities and renal injury from NaP-containing colonoscopy preparations.

4.3 Pregnancy

While the safety of colonoscopy and sigmoidoscopy has been established in the general population, colonoscopy during pregnancy has only been described in small case series and case reports. The main two concerns in performing colonoscopy during pregnancy are maternal and fetal complications including usual complications of colonoscopy, premature delivery, low birth weight, fetal anomalies, placental abruption, fetal compression, medication toxicity, and stillbirth. In a retrospective study by Cappell et al. there were no maternal complications in 48 flexible sigmoidoscopies and 8 colonoscopies performed in pregnant women done during different trimesters (Cappell et al, 1996). Effects of the procedure on vital signs, including oxygen saturation, were clinically and statistically insignificant. Four fetal demises were reported in the study, but all 4 cases occurred in high-risk pregnancies and at least 2 months after the procedure. The group who underwent colonoscopy or sigmoidoscopy had similar outcomes in term of premature delivery, low birth weight, and cesarean section compared to aged-matched pregnant women who did not undergo endoscopy (Cappell et al, 1996). In another retrospective study from the same authors, there were no major maternal complications in 20 pregnant women undergoing colonoscopy. Mild, transient hypotension occurred in 2 patients (Cappell et al, 2010). The colonic preparations in their study included PEG, sodium phosphate, magnesium citrate, and water/saline enemas. Anesthetics and sedative medications that were administered during colonoscopy included meperidine (category B drug during pregnancy), morphine (category C), fentanyl (category C), midazolam (category D), diazepam (category D), propofol (category B), and thiopental (category C). Six patients underwent the procedure without anesthesia. No fetal distress occurred during colonoscopy in the 6 patients who underwent fetal heart rate monitoring. In this study, also, there were no statistical differences between study group and the national average for pregnancy outcomes or a matched group in term of fetal outcomes including involuntary abortion, premature delivery, low birth weight, low Apgar score, cesarean section rate, congenital defects or stillbirth. Despite the estimate that 1500 colonoscopies are done annually during pregnancy in the United States, there are no prospective studies on colonoscopy in pregnancy (Cappell et al, 2010). Based on the aforementioned retrospective studies, it appears that both colonoscopy and sigmoidoscopy are safe in pregnancy. Even though PEG, NaP and magnesium citrate are category C drugs, they were administered for colonoscopy preparation without maternal or fetal complications (Cappell et al, 2010, although our group would strongly advise against the use of NaP containing preparations in these patients). The diagnostic and therapeutic yield for colonoscopy or sigmoidoscopy is highest for rectal bleeding compared to abdominal pain, constipation, or diarrhea (Cappell et al, 1996; Cappell et al, 2010). The safest timing for colonoscopy or sigmoidoscopy during pregnancy is not known, however, sigmoidoscopies were performed almost equally in all three trimesters in the first study while colonoscopies took place primarily in the second trimester in the second study by Cappell, (Cappell et al, 1996; Cappell et al, 2010). The ASGE recommends using PEG-ESL for colonoscopy preparation during pregnancy (Anderson et al, 2009). However, there are no controlled studies on the use and safety of PEG during pregnancy. The ASGE also suggests that colonoscopy should only be performed when the potential benefit outweighs the potential risks. ASGE guidelines for endoscopy in pregnant and lactating women published in 2005 recommend the following: procedures must always have a strong indication, defer to second trimester if possible, use category A or B sedative medications with the lowest effective dose, minimize procedure time, place pregnant patients with a left pelvic tilt or left lateral position. However, these recommendations are based on expert opinions rather than solid evidence based data (Qureshi et al, 2005).

4.4 Low body weight

Lower body mass index (BMI) has been associated with more difficult colonoscopy, lower cecal intubation rate, longer insertion time and more painful colonoscopy (Anderson et al, 2001; Chung et al, 2007); however there are no data regarding if bowel preparation affects these findings. There are also no data to indicate that changes need to be made in the duration of the preparation, timing, and the amount of lavage solutions administered in the preparation for colonoscopy in patients with a low BMI. A pharmacokinetic analysis of liquid NaP colonoscopy preparation performed by our group has demonstrated that lower body weight individuals, particularly females, develop more pronounced hyperphosphatemia, acidosis, and decreased ionized calcium than normal weight or obese individuals when using these preparations (Ehrenpreis, 2009).

4.5 Possible inflammatory bowel disease, ischemic colitis, or non-steroidal anti-inflammatory drug-induced colitis

Colonic mucosal changes that mimic grossly inflammatory bowel disease (IBD) changes or non-steroidal anti-inflammatory drug-induced colitis have been described with NaP preparations. Colonoscopic findings include aphthoid lesions, erosions and ulcers (Rejchrt et al, 2004). Histologically, focal nonspecific inflammation, mucosal erosion, edema of the lamina propria, focal hemorrhage, and ulceration are seen (Rejchrt et al, 2004). In early studies, these mucosal changes were seen in more than 24% of patients who used NaP for bowel preparation (Zwas et al, 1996). More recent studies with a larger number of patients suggest that these changes occur in 3.3% of patients using these preparations (Rejchrt et al, 2004). Due to these potential mucosal changes, AGSE discourages the use of NaP as a bowel cleanser in the initial colonoscopy in patients with a suspicion of IBD (Anderson et al, 2009).

4.6 Diabetus mellitus

Bowel preparation seems to be less effective in diabetic patients. In a study done by Taylor and Schubert, there was a significant difference in the quality of the bowel preparations with PEG ELS between diabetic and non-diabetic patients ($p < 0.001$) (Taylor & Schubert, 2001). Only 62% of the diabetic group had a preparation rated as good or better compared to 97% of the non-diabetic group ($p < 0.001$) (Taylor & Schubert, 2001). In this study, 9% of diabetic patients had a preparation rated as poor or futile, necessitating repeat colonoscopy compared to none in patients without diabetes ($p < 0.01$). Among the diabetic group, there was no difference in bowel preparation between patients on insulin and not on insulin, those with hemoglobin A1c (Hb A1c) values >8% and those with values <8%, and those with and without diabetic neuropathy (Taylor & Schubert, 2001). In another study done by Oztur et al. using NaP as a bowel cleansing agent, optimal bowel cleansing was achieved in 70% diabetics compared to 94%in the non-diabetic group ($P = 0.002$). Among the diabetic patients, there was a significant correlation between the quality of bowel cleansing and HbA1c level, duration of diabetes mellitus, and presence of late complications of diabetes ($P < 0.05$) (Ozturk et al, 2010). Of note, both of the aforementioned studies were small. In a larger study of 362 patients, diabetes was independent predictor of poor bowel cleansing in patients using PEG as the agent for preparation (Chung et al, 2009).

4.7 Colonoscopy preparation in children

Colonoscopy is relatively uncommon in pediatric population. There are no uniform protocols or national guidelines for colonoscopy preparation. PEG ESL is the most common bowel cleansing agent used in pediatrics. However the large volume and potentially unpleasant taste of these solutions has been a major limitation in their use. Placement of a nasogastric tube has been used in some studies. In one study, PEG ESL was better tolerated than total gut irrigation using normal saline with added potassium. Both regimens demonstrated equivalency for side effects and efficacy (Chattopadhyay et al, 2004). PEG-3350 without electrolytes (Miralax) has been increasingly used for bowel cleansing for colonoscopy in children. PEG 3350 solution was first studied with a 4 day regimen, showing safety, efficacy, and tolerability in children (Safder et al, 2008). A subsequent study showed that even a one day regimen of PEG-3350 is effective in 93% of children (Adamiak et al, 2010).

Bisacodyl with NaP enemas has been tested in different studies with a high rate of compliance and bowel preparation. In a study of 98 children between 30 months to 12 years of age, the compliance of the bisacodyl with NaP enema group was 100%, compared to 88% in PEG group. Good to excellent bowel preparation achieved in 95% in bisacodyl with NaP enema group compared to 88% in PEG ESL group (Shaoul & Haloon L, 2007). However, another study of 70 children did not show the same results. PEG ESL was superior for bowel cleansing ($p < 0.0001$) but was inferior to NaP enema in terms of tolerance and compliance ($p < 0.003$) (Dahshan et al, 1999).

Oral NaP was studied for use as a bowel preparation for pediatric colonoscopy. One study showed that NaP was superior to PEG-based solutions in term of tolerance, compliance and bowel cleansing (Gremse et al, 1996). However, there is potential risk of electrolytes and fluid disturbance in NaP. Our group recommends avoidance of these preparations in children.

Magnesium citrate was used combined with senna (X-prep) in some pediatric patients. This combination was shown to be superior to bisacodyl combined with a NaP enema ($p < 0.0001$), but inferior to PEG ELS ($p < 0.075$) in term of quality of bowel cleansing (Dahshan et al, 1999). Overall tolerance and compliance were significantly better than PEG ELS ($p < 0.003$) (Dahshan et al, 1999). In another study, magnesium citrate was used with bisacodyl and demonstrated to be superior to NaP ($P = .013$) in term of bowel cleansing. Both regimens were equivalent for tolerance and compliance (El-Baba et al, 2006). In a third study of 48 children, magnesium citrate was used with a NaP enema for a 3 days protocol and compared to a one day regimen of oral NaP alone (Sabri et al, 2008). Bowel cleansing was similar in two groups (71% good or excellent) and side effects were similar except nausea which was more frequent in NaP. However, patients stated that they were more willing to repeat NaP alone compared to the combination regimen (77%vs 32%, respectively, $P < 0.006$) (Sabri et al, 2008).

5. Conclusion

The choice of bowel preparation for colonoscopy should be individualized after thorough patient screening. Next generation lower volume regimens have been developed that are well tolerated and preferred by the patients over traditional larger volume bowel preparations. NaP preparations are generally more effective and better tolerated than PEG-ELSs. However there is increasing concern regarding toxicity of NaP formulations, especially in light of the availability of newer, potentially better tolerated preparations.

6. Future research

There is ongoing research to develop safe bowel preparation regimens that provide good bowel cleansing along with better patient tolerability and low side effect profile. Further research is also needed for effect of bowel preparations in the elderly, pregnant women and children as well as in patients with significant morbidities. Gender based risk of adverse effects is a newly studied phenomenon that requires additional study.

7. References

Adamiak, T; Altaf, M; Jensen, M.K; Sultan, M; Ramprasad, J; Ciecierega, T; Sherry, K & Miranda, A (2010). One-day bowel preparation with polyethylene glycol 3350: an effective regimen for colonoscopy in children. Gastrointest Endosc, Vol.71, No.3, (Mar 2010), pp.573-7, ISSN: 0016-5107.

Adams, C; Cardwell, C; Cook, C; Edwards, R; Atkin, W.S & Morton, D.G (2003). Effect of hysterectomy status on polyp detection rates at screening flexible sigmoidoscopy. Gastrointest Endosc, Vol.57, No.7, (Jun 2003), pp.848-53, ISSN: 0016-5107.

Ainley, E.J; Winwood, P.J & Begley, J.P (2005). Measurement of serum electrolytes and phosphate after sodium phosphate colonoscopy bowel preparation: an evaluation. Dig Dis Sci, Vol.50, No.7, (2005), pp.1319-23, ISSN: 0163-2116.

American Society for Gastrointestinal Endoscopy. (2000). Appropriate use of gastrointestinal endoscopy. *Gastrointestinal endoscopy*. Vol.52, No.6, (2000), pp.831-837, ISSN: 0016-5107.

Anderson, J.C; Messina, C.R; Cohn, W; Gottfried, E; Ingber, S; Bernstein, G; Coman, E & Polito, J (2001). Factors predictive of difficult colonoscopy. Gastrointest Endosc, Vol.54, No.5, (Nov 2001), pp.558-62, ISSN: 0016-5107.

Anderson, M.A; Ben-Menachem, T; Gan, S.I; Appalaneni, V; Banerjee, S; Cash, B.D; Fisher, L; Harrison, M.E; Fanelli, R.D; Fukami, N; Ikenberry, S.O; Jain, R; Khan, K; Krinsky, M.L; Lichtenstein, D.R; Maple, J.T; Shen, B; Strohmeyer, L; Baron, T & Dominitz, J.A (2009). ASGE Standards of Practice Committee. Management of antithrombotic agents for endoscopic procedures. Gastrointest Endosc, Vol.70, No.6, (Dec 2009), pp.1060-70, ISSN: 0016-5107.

Aronchick, CA; Lipshutz, WH; Wright, SH; Dufrayne, F & Bergman, G. (2000).A novel tableted purgative for colonoscopic preparation: efficacy and safety comparisons with Colyte and Fleet Phospho-Soda. *Gastrointest Endosc*,Vol.52, No.3, (Sep 2000),pp.346-52, ISSN: 0016-5107.

Bac, D.J; van Blankenstein, M; de Marie, S & Fieren, M.W (1994). Peritonitis following endoscopic polypectomy in a peritoneal dialysis patient: the need for antibiotic prophylaxis. Infection, Vol.22, No.3, (May-Jun 1994), pp.220-1, ISSN: 0163-4453

Banerjee, S; Shen, B; Baron, T.H; Nelson, D.B; Anderson, M.A; Cash, B.D; Dominitz, J.A; Gan, S.I; Harrison, M.E; Ikenberry, S.O; Jagannath, S.B; Lichtenstein, D; Fanelli, R.D; Lee, K; van Guilder, T & Stewart, L.E (2008). ASGE STANDARDS OF PRACTICE COMMITTEE. Antibiotic prophylaxis for GI endoscopy. Gastrointest Endosc, Vol. 67, No. 6, (May 2008), pp. 791-8, ISSN: 0016-5107.

Belsey, J; Epstein, O & Heresbach, D. (2007).Systematic review: oral bowel preparation for colonoscopy. *Aliment Pharmacol Ther*,Vol.25,(2007),pp.373-84, ISSN: 0269-2813.

Beloosesky, Y; Grinblat, J; Weiss, A; Grosman, B; Gafter, U & Chagnac, A (2003). Electrolyte disorders following oral sodium phosphate administration for bowel cleansing in elderly patients. Arch Intern Med, Vol.163, No.7, (2003), pp.803-8, ISSN: 0003-9926 (print); 1538-3679 (online).

Bhanji, S; Williams, B; Sheller, B; Elwood, T & Mancl, L (2002). Transient bacteremia induced by toothbrushing a comparison of the Sonicare toothbrush with a conventional toothbrush. Pediatr Dent, Vol.24, No.4, (Jul-Aug 2002), pp.295-9, ISSN: 0164-1263.

Calderwood, A.H. & Jacobson, B.C. (2010). Comprehensive validation of the Boston Bowel Preparation Scale. *Gastrointest Endosc*, Vol. 72, No. 4, (October 2010), pp. 682-92, ISSN: 0016-5107

Cappell, M.S; Colon, V.J & Sidhom, O.A (1996). A study at 10 medical centers of the safety and efficacy of 48 flexible sigmoidoscopies and 8 colonoscopies during pregnancy with follow-up of fetal outcome and with comparison to control groups. Dig Dis Sci, Vol.41, No.12, (Dec 1996), pp.2353-61, ISSN: 0163-2116.

Cappell, M.S; Fox, S.R & Gorrepati, N (2010). Safety and efficacy of colonoscopy during pregnancy: an analysis of pregnancy outcome in 20 patients. J Reprod Med, Vol.55, No.3-4, (Mar-Apr 2010), pp.115-23, ISSN: 0024-7758.

Chang, KJ; Erickson, RA; Schandler, S; Coye, T & Moody, C. (1991). Per-rectal pulsed irrigation versus per-oral colonic lavage for colonoscopy preparation: a randomized, controlled trial. *Gastrointest Endosc*, Vol.37, No.4,(Jul-Aug 1991) pp.444-8, ISSN: 0016-5107.

Chattopadhyay, A; Prakash, B; Vepakomma, D; Nagendhar, Y & Vijayakumar (2004). A prospective comparison of two regimes of bowel preparation for pediatric colorectal procedures: normal saline with added potassium vs. polyethylene glycol. Pediatr Surg Int, Vol.20, No.2, (Feb 2004), pp.127-9, ISSN: 0179-0358 (print); 1437-9813 (online).

Chung, Y.W; Han, D.S; Yoo, K.S & Park, C.K (2007). Patient factors predictive of pain and difficulty during sedation-free colonoscopy: a prospective study in Korea. Dig Liver Dis, Vol.39, No.9, (Sep 2007), pp.872-6, ISSN: 1590-8658 (Print); 1878-3562 (online).

Chung, Y.W; Han, D.S; Park, K.H; Kim, K.O; Park, C.H; Hahn, T; Yoo, K.S; Park, S.H; Kim, J.H & Park, C.K (2009). Patient factors predictive of inadequate bowel preparation using polyethylene glycol: a prospective study in Korea. J Clin Gastroenterol, Vol.43, No.5, (May-Jun 2009), pp.448-52, ISSN: 0192-0790 (print); 1539-2031 (online).

Church JM (1994). Complete colonoscopy: how often? And if not, why not? Am J Gastroenterol, Vol.89, No.4, (Apr 1994), pp.556-60, ISSN: 0002-9270 9print); 1572-0241 (online).

Church, JM. (1998).Effectiveness of polyethylene glycol antegrade gut lavage bowel preparation for colonoscopy. Timing is the key! *Dis Colon Rectum,* Vol.41,(1998), pp.1223-5, ISSN: 00123706.

Clark, L.E & DiPalma, J.A. (2004). Safety issues regarding colonic cleansing for diagnostic and surgical procedures. *Drug Saf,* Vol. 27, No. 15, (2004), pp. 1235-42. ISSN: 0114-5916

Cornelius, L.K; Reddix, R.N & Jr, Carpenter, J.L (2003). Periprosthetic knee joint infection following colonoscopy. A case report. J Bone Joint Surg Am, Vol.85-A, No.12, (Dec 2003), pp.2434-6, ISSN: 0021-9355.

Dahshan, A; Lin, C.H; Peters, J; Thomas, R & Tolia, V (1999). A randomized, prospective study to evaluate the efficacy and acceptance of three bowel preparations for colonoscopy in children. Am J Gastroenterol, Vol.94, No.12, (Dec 1999), pp.3497-501, ISSN: 0002-9270 (print); 1572-0241 (online).

Delegge, M & Kaplan, R. (2005). Efficacy of bowel preparation with the use of a prepackaged, low fibre diet with a low sodium, magnesium citrate cathartic vs. a clear liquid diet with a standard sodium phosphate cathartic. *Aliment Pharmacol Ther,* Vol.21, No.12, (Jun 2005), pp.1491-5, ISSN: 0269-2813.

Desmeules, S; Bergeron, M.J & Isenring, P (2003). Acute phosphate nephropathy and renal failure. N Engl J Med, Vol.309, (2003), pp.1006, ISSN: 0028-4793 (print); 1533-4406 (online).

DiPalma, JA & Marshall, JB. (1990).Comparison of a new sulfate-free polyethylene glycol electrolyte lavage solution versus a standard solution for colonoscopy cleansing. *Gastrointest Endosc,*Vol.36, No.3, (May-Jun 1990), pp.285-9, ISSN: 0016-5107.

DiPalma, JA; Wolff, BG; Meagher, A & Cleveland, M. (2003).Comparison of reduced volume versus four liters sulfate-free electrolyte lavage solutions for colonoscopy colon cleansing. *Am J Gastroenterol,*Vol.98, No.10, (Oct 2003), pp.2187-91, ISN: 0002-9270.

Ehrenpreis, ED; Nogueras, JJ; Botoman, VA; Bonner, GF; Zaitman, D & Secrest, KM. (1996). Serum electrolyte abnormalities secondary to Fleet's Phospho-Soda colonoscopy prep. *Surg Endosc,* Vol.10, (1996),pp.1022-24, ISSN: 0930-2794.

Ehrenpreis, E.D.; Wieland, J.M.; Cabral, J.; Estevez, V.; Zaitman, D. & Secrest, K. (1997). Symptomatic hypocalcemia, hypomagnesemia, and hyperphosphatemia secondary to Fleet's Phospho-Soda colonoscopy preparation in a patient with a jejunoileal bypass. *Dig Dis Sci.* Vol. 42, No. 4, (April 1997), pp. 858-60, ISSN: 0163-2116

Ehrenpreis, E.D. (2009). Increased serum phosphate levels and calcium fluxes are seen in smaller individuals after a single dose of sodium phosphate colon cleansing solution: a pharmacokinetic analysis. *Aliment Pharmacol Ther.* Vol. 29, No. 11, (June 2009), pp. 1202-11, ISSN: 1365-2036

El-Baba, M.F; Padilla, M; Houston, C; Madani, S; Lin, C.H; Thomas, R & Tolia, V (2006). A prospective study comparing oral sodium phosphate solution to a bowel cleansing preparation with nutrition food package in children. J Pediatr Gastroenterol Nutr, Vol.42, No.2, (Feb 2006), pp.174-7, ISSN: 0277-2116 9print); 1536-4801 (online).

Ell, C; Fischbach, W; Bronisch, HJ; Dertinger, S; Layer, P; Rünzi, M; Schneider, T; Kachel, G; Grüger, J; Köllinger, M; Nagell, W; Goerg, KJ; Wanitschke, R & Gruss, HJ.

(2008).Randomized trial of low-volume PEG solution versus standard PEG + electrolytes for bowel cleansing before colonoscopy. *Am J Gastroenterol*,Vol.103, No.4, (Apr 2008), pp.883-93, ISN: 0002-9270.

El Sayed, AM; Kanafani, ZA; Mourad, FH; Soweid, AM; Barada, KA; Adorian, CS, Nasreddine, WA & Sharara, AI. (2003). A randomized single-blind trial of whole versus split-dose polyethylene glycol-electrolyte solution for colonoscopy preparation. *Gastrointest Endosc*,Vol.58, (2003), pp.36-40, ISSN: 0016-5107.

Food and Drug Administration. (December, 2008). Oral Sodium Phosphate (OSP) Products for Bowel Cleansing (marketed as Visicol and OsmoPrep, and oral sodium phosphate products available without a prescription). In: Food and Drug Administration, 3/15/2011, available from http://www.fda.gov/Drugs/DrugSafety/PostmarketDrugSafetyInformationforPatientsandProviders/ucm103354.htm

Froehlich, F; Wietlisbach, V; Gonvers, JJ; Burnand, B & Vader, JP. (2005).Impact of colonic cleansing on quality and diagnostic yield of colonoscopy: the European Panel of Appropriateness of Gastrointestinal Endoscopy European multicenter study. *Gastrointest Endosc*,Vol.61, No.3, (Mar 2005), pp.378-84, ISSN: 0016-5107.

Frommer, D. (1997). Cleansing ability and tolerance of three bowel preparations for colonoscopy. *Dis Colon Rectum*,Vol.40, (1997), pp.100-4, ISSN: 00123706.

Goldman, G.D; Miller, S.A; Furman, D.S; et al (1985). Does bacteremia occur during flexible sigmoidoscopy? Am J Gastroenterol, Vol.80, (1985), pp.621-3, ISSN: 0002-9270.

Gremse, D.A; Sacks, A.I & Raines, S (1996). Comparison of oral sodium phosphate to polyethylene glycol-based solution for bowel preparation for colonoscopy in children. J Pediatr Gastroenterol Nutr, Vol.23, No.5, (Dec 1996), pp.586-90, ISSN: 0277-2116 (print); 1536-4801 (online).

Grossman, E.B; Maranino, A.N; Zamora, D.C; et al (2010). Antiplatelet medications increase the risk of post-polypectomy bleeding. Gastrointest Endosc, Vol.71, (2010), pp.AB138, ISSN: 0016-5107.

Gumurdulu, Y; Serin, E; Ozer, B; Gokcel, A & Boyacioglu, S (2004). Age as a predictor of hyperphosphatemia after oral phosphosoda administration for colon preparation. J Gastroenterol Hepatol, Vol.19, No.1, (2004), pp.68-72, ISSN: 0815-9319 9print); 1440-1746 (online).

Harewood, GC; Sharma, VK & de Garmo, P. (2003). Impact of colonoscopy preparation quality on detection of suspected colonic neoplasia. *Gastrointest Endosc*,Vol.58, No.1, (Jul 2003), pp.76-9,. ISSN: 0016-5107.

Ho, J.M; Juurlink, D.N & Cavalcanti, R.B (2010). Hypokalemia following polyethylene glycol-based bowel preparation for colonoscopy in older hospitalized patients with significant comorbidities. Ann Pharmacother, Vol.44, No.3, (Mar 2010), pp.466-70, ISSN: 1060-0280 (print); 1542-6270 (online).

Hui, A.J; Wong, R.M; Ching, J.Y; Hung, L.C, Chung, S.C & Sung, J.J (2004). Risk of colonoscopic polypectomy bleeding with anticoagulants and antiplatelet agents: analysis of 1657 cases. Gastrointest Endosc, Vol.59, No.1, (Jan 2004), pp.44-8, ISSN: 0016-5107.

Iakovou, I; Schmidt, T; Bonizzoni, E; Ge, L; Sangiorgi, G.M; Stankovic, G; Airoldi, F; Chieffo, A; Montorfano, M; Carlino, M; Michev, I; Corvaja, N; Briguori, C; Gerckens, U; Grube, E & Colombo, A (2005). Incidence, predictors, and outcome of thrombosis after successful implantation of drug-eluting stents. JAMA, Vol.293, No.17, (May 2005), pp.2126-30, ISSN: 00987484 (print); 15383598 (online).

Iida, Y.; Miura, S.; Asada, Y.; Fukuoka, K.; Toya, D.; Tanaka, N. & Fujisawa, M. (1992). Bowel preparation for the total colonoscopy by 2000 ml of balanced lavage solution (GoLytely) and sennoside. *Gastroenterol Jpn*, Vol. 27, No. 6, (December 1992), pp. 728-33, ISSN: 0944-1174

Johanson, JF; Popp, JW Jr; Cohen, LB; Lottes, SR; Forbes, WP; Walker, K; Carter, E;, Zhang, B & Rose, M. (2007).A randomized, multicenter study comparing the safety and efficacy of sodium phosphate tablets with 2L polyethylene glycol solution plus bisacodyl tablets for colon cleansing. *Am J Gastroenterol*,Vol.102, No.10, (Oct 2007), pp.2238-46, ISN: 0002-9270.

Kazarian, ES; Carreira, FS; Toribara, NW & Denberg, TD. (2008).Colonoscopy completion in a large safety net health care system. *Clin Gastroenterol Hepatol*,Vol.6, No.4, (April 2008), pp.377-8, ISSN: 1542-3565.

King, S.B 3rd; Smith, S.C Jr; Hirshfeld, J.W Jr; Jacobs, A.K; Morrison, D.A; Williams, D.O; Feldman, T.E; Kern, M.J; O'Neill, W.W; Schaff, H.V & Whitlow, P.L; ACC/AHA/SCAI, Adams, C.D; Anderson, J.L; Buller, C.E; Creager, M.A; Ettinger, S.M; Halperin, J.L; Hunt, S.A; Krumholz, H.M; Kushner, F.G; Lytle, B.W; Nishimura, R; Page, R.L; Riegel, B; Tarkington, L.G & Yancy, C.W (2008). 2007 focused update of the ACC/AHA/SCAI 2005 guideline update for percutaneous coronary intervention: a report of the American College of Cardiology/American Heart Association Task Force on Practice guidelines. J Am Coll Cardiol. 2008 Jan 15;51(2):172-209. ISSN: 0735-1097

Kontani, M; Hara, A; Ohta, S & Ikeda, T (2005). Hypermagnesaemia induced by massive cathartic ingestion in an elderly woman without pre-existing renal dysfunction. Intern Med, Vol.44, (2005), pp.448, ISSN: 0918-2918 (Print); 1349-7235 (online).

Lagares-Garcia, J.A; Kurek, S; Collier, B; Diaz, F; Schilli, R; Richey, J & Moore, R.A (2001). Colonoscopy in octogenarians and older patients. Surg Endosc, Vol.15, No.3, (Mar 2001), pp.262-5, ISSN: 1432-2218 (online).

Lai, E.J.; Calderwood, A.H.; Doros, G.; Fix, O.K. & Jacobson, B.C. (2009). The Boston bowel preparation scale: a valid and reliable instrument for colonoscopy-oriented research. *Gastrointest Endosc*, Vol. 69, No. 3, (March 2009), pp. 620-25, ISSN: 0016-5107

Levin, B; Lieberman, DA; McFarland, B; Andrews, KS; Brooks, D; Bond, J; Dash, C; Giardiello, FM; Glick, S; Johnson, D; Johnson, CD; Levin, TR; Pickhardt, PJ; Rex, DK; Smith, RA; Thorson, A; Winawer, SJ; American Cancer Society Colorectal Cancer Advisory Group; US Multi-Society Task Force & American College of Radiology Colon Cancer Committee. (2008). Screening and surveillance for the early detection of colorectal cancer and adenomatous polyps, 2008: a joint guideline from the American Cancer Society, the US Multi-Society Task Force on Colorectal Cancer, and the American College of Radiology.*CA Cancer J Clin*,Vol.58, No.3, (May-Jun 2008),pp.130-60, Online ISSN: 1542-4863.

Levy, M.J; Norton, I.D; Clain, J.E; et al (2007). Prospective study of bacteremia and complications with EUS FNA of rectal and perirectal lesions. Clin Gastroenterol Hepatol, Vol.5, (2007), pp.684-9, ISSN: 1542-3565.

Lichtenstein, G. (2009).Bowel preparations for colonoscopy: a review. *Am J Health Syst Pharm,Vol.*66, No.1, (Jan 2009), pp.27-37, ISSN: 1079-2082.

Li, P.K; Szeto, C.C; Piraino, B; Bernardini, J; Figueiredo, A.E; Gupta, A; Johnson, D.W; Kuijper, E.J; Lye, W.C; Salzer, W; Schaefer, F & Struijk, D.G (2010). Peritoneal dialysis-related infections recommendations: 2010 update. Perit Dial Int, Vol.30, No.4, (Jul-Aug 2010), pp.393-423, ISSN: 0896-8608 (print); 1718-4304 (online).

Llach, J; Elizalde, J.I; Bordas, J.M; et al (1999). Prospective assessment of the risk of bacteremia in cirrhotic patients undergoing lower intestinal endoscopy. Gastrointest Endosc, Vol.49, (1999), pp.214-7, ISSN: 0016-5107.

Lockhart, P.B; Brennan, M.T; Sasser, H.C; Fox, P.C; Paster, B.J & Bahrani-Mougeot, F.K (2008). Bacteremia associated with tooth brushing and dental extraction. Circulation. Vol.117, No.24, (Jun 2008), pp.3118-25, ISSN: 0009-7322.

Lukens, F.J; Loeb, D.S; Machicao, V.I; Achem, S.R & Picco, M.F (2002). Colonoscopy in octogenarians: a prospective outpatient study. Am J Gastroenterol, Vol.97, No.7, (2002), pp.1722-5, ISSN: 0002-9270 (print); 1572-0241(online).

Marschall, H.U & Bartels F (1998). Life-threatening complications of nasogastric administration of polyethylene glycol-electrolyte solution (Golytely) for bowel cleansing. Gastrointest Endosc, Vol.47, No.5, (1998), pp.408-10, ISSN: 0016-5107.

Nelson, D.B (2003). Infectious disease complications of GI endoscopy: part I, endogenous infections. Gastrointest Endosc, Vol.57, (2003), pp.546-56, ISSN: 0016-5107.

Ness, R.M; Manam, R; Hoen, H & Chalasani, N (2001). Predictors of inadequate bowel preparation for colonoscopy. Am J Gastroenterol, Vol.96, (2001), pp.1797, ISSN: 0002-9270 (print); 1572-0241 (online).

Ozturk, N.A; Gokturk, H.S; Demir, M; Unler, G.K; Gur, G & Yilmaz, U (2010). Efficacy and safety of sodium phosphate for colon cleansing in type 2 diabetes mellitus. South Med J, Vol.103, No.11, (Nov 2010), pp.1097-102, ISSN: 0038-4348 (print); 1541-8243 (online).

Parakkal, D. & Ehrenpreis E.D. (2010). Calcium phosphate nephropathy from colonoscopy preparations: effect of body weight. *Am J Gastroenterol,* Vol.105, No.3, (Mar 2010), pp. 705, ISSN: 0002-9270

Pelham, R.W.; Russell, R.G.; Padgett, E.L.; Reno, F.E. & Cleveland, M. (2009). Safety of oral sulfates in rats and dogs contrasted with phosphate-induced nephropathy in rats. *Int J Toxicol,* Vol. 28, No. 2, (March-April 2009), pp.99-112, ISSN: 1091-5818

Piraino, B; Bailie, G.R; Bernardini, J; Boeschoten, E; Gupta, A; Holmes, C; Kuijper, E.J; Li, P.K; Lye, W.C; Mujais, S; Paterson, D.L; Fontan, M.P; Ramos, A; Schaefer, F & Uttley, L; ISPD Ad Hoc Advisory Committee (2005). Peritoneal dialysis-related infections recommendations: 2005 update. Perit Dial Int, Vol.25, No.2, (Mar-Apr 2005), pp.107-31, ISSN: 0896-8608 (print); 1718-4304 (online).

Qureshi, A; Ismail, S; Azmi, A; Murugan, P & Husin, M (2000). Poor bowel preparation in patients undergoing colonoscopy. Med J Malaysia, Vol.55, No.2, (Jun 2000), pp.246-8, ISSN: 0300-5283.

Qureshi, W.A; Rajan, E; Adler, D.G; Davila, R.E; Hirota, W.K; Jacobson, B.C; Leighton, J.A; Zuckerman, M.J; Hambrick, R.D; Fanelli, R.D; Baron, T & Faigel, D.O (2005); American Society for Gastrointestinal Endoscopy. ASGE Guideline: Guidelines for endoscopy in pregnant and lactating women. Gastrointest Endosc, Vol.61, No.3, (Mar 2005), pp.357-62, ISSN: 0016-5107.

Ray, S.M; Piraino, B & Holley, J (1990). Peritonitis following colonoscopy in a peritoneal dialysis patient. Perit Dial Int, Vol.10, No.1, (1990), pp.97-8, ISSN: 0896-8608; 1718-4304 (online).

Reilly, T & Walker, G (2004). Reasons for poor colonic preparation with inpatients. Gastroenterol Nurs, Vol.27, No.3, (May-Jun 2004), pp.115-7, ISSN: 1042-895X; 1538-9766 (online).

Rejchrt, S.; Bures, J.; Siroký, M.; Kopácová, M.; Slezák, L. & Langr, F. (2004). A prospective, observational study of colonic mucosal abnormalities associated with orally administered sodium phosphate for colon cleansing before colonoscopy. *Gastrointest Endosc*, Vol. 59, No. 6, (May 2004), pp.651-4, ISSN: 0016-5107.

Rex, DK; Imperiale, TF; Latinovich, DR & Bratcher, LL. (2002).Impact of bowel preparation on efficiency and cost of colonoscopy. *Am J Gastroenterol*,Vol.97, No.7, (Jul 2002), pp.1696-700, ISN: 0002-9270.

A)Rex, D.K.; Petrini, J.L.; Baron, T.H.; Chak, A.; Cohen, J.; Deal, S.E.; Hoffman, B.; Jacobson, B.C.; Mergener, K.; Petersen, B.T.; Safdi, M.A.; Faigel, D.O.; Pike, I.M. & ASGE/ACG Taskforce on Quality in Endoscopy. (2006). Quality indicators for colonoscopy. *Am J Gastroenterol*, Vol. 101, No. 4, (April 2006), pp. 873–85, ISN: 0002-9270

B)Rex, DK; Schwartz, H; Goldstein, M; Popp, J; Katz, S; Barish, C; Karlstadt, RG; Rose, M; Walker, K; Lottes, S; Ettinger, N & Zhang, B. (2006).Safety and colon-cleansing efficacy of a new residue-free formulation of sodium phosphate tablets. *Am J Gastroenterol*,Vol.101, No.11, (Nov 2006), pp.2594-604, ISSN: 0002-9270.

Rex, DK; Johnson, DA; Anderson, JC; Schoenfeld, PS; Burke, CA; Inadomi, JM & American College of Gastroenterology. (2009).American College of Gastroenterology guidelines for colorectal cancer screening 2009 [corrected]. *Am J Gastroenterol*,Vol.104, No.3,(Mar 2009),pp.739-50, ISSN: 0002-9270

Rex, DK; Di Palma, JA; Rodriguez, R; McGowan, J & Cleveland, M. (2010).A randomized clinical study comparing reduced-volume oral sulfate solution with standard 4-liter sulfate-free electrolyte lavage solution as preparation for colonoscopy. *Gastrointest Endosc*,Vol.72, (2010), pp.328-336, ISSN: 0016-5107.

Sabri, M; Di Lorenzo, C; Henderson, W; Thompson, W; Barksdale, E Jr & Khan, S (2008). Colon cleansing with oral sodium phosphate in adolescents: dose, efficacy, acceptability, and safety. Am J Gastroenterol, Vol.103, No.6, (Jun 2008), pp.1533-9, ISSN: 0002-9270 (print); 1572-0241 (online).

Safder, S; Demintieva, Y; Rewalt, M & Elitsur, Y (2008). Stool consistency and stool frequency are excellent clinical markers for adequate colon preparation after polyethylene glycol 3350 cleansing protocol: a prospective clinical study in children. Gastrointest Endosc, Vol.68, No.6, (Dec 2008), pp.1131-5, ISSN: 0016-5107.

Saunders, B.P; Fukumoto, M; Halligan, S; Jobling, C; Moussa, M.E; Bartram, C.I & Williams, C.B (1996). Why is colonoscopy more difficult in women? Gastrointest Endosc, Vol.43, No.2 pt 1, (Feb 1996), pp.124-6, ISSN: 0016-5107.

Schelling, J.R. (2000). Fatal hypermagnesemia. *Clin Nephrol*, Vol. 53, No. 1, (January 2000), pp. 61-5, ISSN: 0301-0430.

Seeff, L.C; Richards, T.B; Shapiro, J.A; et al (2004). How many endoscopies are performed for colorectal cancer screening? Results from CDC's survey of endoscopic capacity. Gastroenterology, Vol.127, (2004), pp.1670-7, ISSN: 0016-5085.

Seinela, L; Pehkonen, E; Laasanen, T & Ahvenainen, J (2003). Bowel preparation for colonoscopy in very old patients: a randomized prospective trial comparing oral sodium phosphate and polyethylene glycol electrolyte lavage solution. Scand J Gastroenterol, Vol.38, No.2, (2003), pp.216-20, ISSN: 0036-5521 (Print); 1502-7708 (online).

Shah, S.G; Brooker, J.C; Thapar, C; Williams, C.B & Saunders, B.P (2002). Patient pain during colonoscopy: an analysis using real-time magnetic endoscope imaging. Endoscopy, Vol.34, No.6, (Jun 2002), pp.435-40, ISSN: 0013-726X (Print); 1438-8812 (online).

Shaoul, R & Haloon, L (2007). An assessment of bisacodyl-based bowel preparation for colonoscopy in children. J Gastroenterol, Vol.42, No.1, (Jan 2007), pp.26-8, ISSN: 0944-1174 (Print); 1435-5922 (online).

Sharma, VK; Chockalingham, SK; Ugheoke, EA; Kapur, A; Ling, PH; Vasudeva, R & Howden, CW. (1998).Prospective, randomized, controlled comparison of the use of polyethylene glycol electrolyte lavage solution in four-liter versus two-liter volumes and pretreatment with either magnesium citrate or bisacodyl for colonoscopy preparation. *Gastrointest Endosc*,Vol.47, No.2, (Feb 1998), pp.167-71, ISSN: 0016-5107.

Singh, M; Mehta, N; Murthy, U.K; Kaul, V; Arif, A & Newman, N (2010). Postpolypectomy bleeding in patients undergoing colonoscopy on uninterrupted clopidogrel therapy. Gastrointest Endosc, Vol.71, No.6, (May 2010), pp.998-1005, ISSN: 0016-5107.

Tan, JJ & Tjandra, JJ. (2006).Which is the optimal bowel preparation for colonoscopy: a meta-analysis. *Colorectal Dis*,Vol.8, (2006), pp.247-58, ISSN 1462-8910.

Taylor, C & Schubert, M.L (2001). Decreased efficacy of polyethylene glycol lavage solution (golytely) in the preparation of diabetic patients for outpatient colonoscopy: a prospective and blinded study. Am J Gastroenterol, Vol.96, No.3, (Mar 2001), pp.710-4, ISSN: 0002-9270 (print); 1572-0241 (online).

Thomas-Gibson, S; Rogers, P; Cooper, S; Man, R; Rutter, MD; Suzuki, N; Swain, D; Thuraisingam, A & Atkin, W. (2006).Judgement of the quality of bowel preparation at screening flexible sigmoidoscopy is associated with variability in adenoma detection rates. *Endoscopy*,Vol.38, No.5, (May 2006), pp.456-60, ISSN: 0013726X.

Thomson, A; Naidoo, P & Crotty, B (1996). Bowel preparation for colonoscopy: a randomized prospective trial comparing sodium phosphate to polyethylene glycol in predominantly elderly population. J Gastroenterol Hepatol, Vol.11, (1996), pp.103-7, ISSN: 0815-9319 (print); 1440-1746 (online).

Ure, T; Dehghan, K; Vernava, A.M 3rd; Longo, W.E; Andrus, C.A & Daniel, G.L (1995). Colonoscopy in the elderly. Low risk, high yield. Surg Endosc, Vol.9, No.5, (May 1995), pp.505-8, ISSN: 1432-2218 (online).

Vanderhooft, J.E & Robinson, R.P (1994). Late infection of a bipolar prosthesis following endoscopy. A case report. J Bone Joint Surg Am, Vol.76, (1994), pp.744-6, ISSN: 0021-9355.

Van der Meer, J.T; Thompson, J; Valkenburg, H.A & Michel, M.F (1992). Epidemiology of bacterial endocarditis in The Netherlands. II. Antecedent procedures and use of prophylaxis. Arch Intern Med, Vol.152, No.9, (Sep 1992), pp.1869-73, ISSN: 0003-9926 (print);1538-3679 (online).

Vanner, SJ; MacDonald, PH; Paterson, WG; Prentice, RS; Da Costa, LR & Beck, IT. (1990).A randomized prospective trial comparing oral sodium phosphate with standard polyethylene glycol-based lavage solution (Golytely) in the preparation of patients for colonoscopy. *Am J Gastroenterol*,Vol.85, No.4, (Apr 1990), pp.422-7, ISSN: 0002-9270.

Wexner, SD. (1996).Preoperative preparation prior to colorectal surgery. *Gastrointest Endosc*,Vol.43, (1996), pp.530-1, ISSN: 0016-5107.

Wexner, S.D.; Beck, D.E.; Baron, T.H.; Fanelli, R.D.; Hyman, N.; Shen, B.; Wasco, K.E. & American Society of Colon and Rectal Surgeons; American Society for Gastrointestinal Endoscopy & Society of American Gastrointestinal and Endoscopic Surgeons. (2006). A consensus document on bowel preparation before colonoscopy: prepared by a task force from the American Society of Colon and Rectal Surgeons (ASCRS), the American Society for Gastrointestinal Endoscopy (ASGE), and the Society of American Gastrointestinal and Endoscopic Surgeons (SAGES). *Gastrointest Endosc*,Vol. 63, No. 7, (Jun 2006), pp. 894-909, ISSN: 0016-5107

Wilson, W; Taubert, K.A; Gewitz, M; Lockhart, P.B; Baddour, L.M; Levison, M; Bolger, A; Cabell, C.H; Takahashi, M; Baltimore, R.S; Newburger, J.W; Strom, B.L; Tani, L.Y; Gerber, M; Bonow, R.O; Pallasch, T; Shulman, S.T; Rowley, A.H; Burns, J.C; Ferrieri, P; Gardner, T; Goff, D & Durack, D.T (2007); American Heart Association Rheumatic Fever, Endocarditis, and Kawasaki Disease Committee; American Heart Association Council on Cardiovascular Disease in the Young; American Heart Association Council on Clinical Cardiology; American Heart Association Council on Cardiovascular Surgery and Anesthesia; Quality of Care and Outcomes Research Interdisciplinary Working Group. Prevention of infective endocarditis: guidelines from the American Heart Association: a guideline from the American Heart Association Rheumatic Fever, Endocarditis, and Kawasaki Disease Committee, Council on Cardiovascular Disease in the Young, and the Council on Clinical Cardiology, Council on Cardiovascular Surgery and Anesthesia, and the Quality of Care and Outcomes Research Interdisciplinary Working Group. Circulation, Vol.116, No.15, (Oct 2007), pp.1736-54, ISSN: 0009-7322.

Worthington, J; Thyssen, M; Chapman, G; Chapman, R & Geraint, M. (2008).A randomised controlled trial of a new 2 litre polyethylene glycol solution versus sodium picosulphate + magnesium citrate solution for bowel cleansing prior to colonoscopy. *Curr Med Res Opin*,Vol.24, Nov.2, (Feb 2008), pp.481-8, ISSN 0300-7995.

Wruble, L; Demicco, M; Medoff, J; Safdi, A; Bernstein, J; Dalke, D; Rose, M; Karlstadt, RG; Ettinger, N & Zhang, B. (2007).Residue-free sodium phosphate tablets (OsmoPrep) versus Visicol for colon cleansing: a randomized, investigator-blinded trial. *Gastrointest Endosc*,Vol.65, No.4,(Apr 2007), pp.660-70, ISSN: 0016-5107.

Ziegenhagen, D.J.; Zehnter, E.; Tacke, W.; Gheorghiu, T. & Krius.W. (1992). Senna versus bisacodyl in addition to GoLytely lavage for colonoscopy preparation: A prospective randomized trial. *Z Gastroenterol* , Vol. 30, No. 1, (January 1992), pp. 17-9, ISSN: 0044-2771.

Zuckerman, M.J; Hirota, W.K; Adler, D.G; Davila, R.E; Jacobson, B.C; Leighton, J.A; Qureshi, W.A; Rajan, E; Hambrick, R.D; Fanelli, R.D; Baron, T.H & Faigel, D.O; Standards of Practice Committee of the American Society for Gastrointestinal Endoscopy (2005).

ASGE guideline: the management of low-molecular-weight heparin and nonaspirin antiplatelet agents for endoscopic procedures. Gastrointest Endosc, Vol.61, No.2, (Feb 2005), pp.189-94, ISSN: 0016-5107.

Zwas, F.R; Cirillo, N.W,; el-Serag, H.B & Eisen, R.N (1996). Colonic mucosal abnormalities associated with oral sodium phosphate solution. Gastrointest Endosc, Vol.43, No.5, (May 1996), pp.463-6, ISSN: 0016-5107.

3

Optimal Bowel Preparation for Colonoscopy

Sansrita Nepal[1], Ashish Atreja[2] and Bret A Lashner[2]
[1]Medicine Institute, Cleveland Clinic
[2]Digestive Diseases Institute, Cleveland Clinic
USA

1. Introduction

Colorectal cancer is the third most cancer in the US and the second most cause of cancer deaths. The general lifetime risk of developing cancer in the United States is about 6%. Colorectal cancer almost always develops from precancerous polyps (abnormal growths) in the colon or rectum. There are various screening tests available for the colon cancer. High sensitivity FOBT, flexible sigmoidoscopy and colonoscopy are the most commonly used ones. Flexible sigmoidoscopy only checks for polyps or cancer inside the rectum and lower third of the colon, while colonoscopy also checks for colon polyps or cancer inside the rectum and the entire colon. It is also used as a follow-up test if anything unusual is found during one of the other screening tests. Other screening tests being studied are virtual colonoscopy and stool DNA test- though currently these are not covered uniformly by the insurance companies.

Colonoscopy is a very important screening test that is thought to be playing a pivotal role in the decline of the colorectal cancer rates in the developed countries by facilitating the early detection and the removal of the adenomatous polyps. Guidelines from national societies recommend routine screening for colorectal cancer starting the age of 50 years in patients at average risk. Adequate bowel preparation is important in assuring the quality and accuracy of the colonoscopy (see figure 1). However, preparing for a colonoscopy can be frustrating for the patients. It is the role of the care providers to take time to explain to the patients how exactly they should approach in order to avoid any failures and repeat exams which can be agonizing for the patient. Regardless of the preparation selected, the potential financial burden of a repeat colonoscopy and preparation can be huge. Specifically, the patient may be required to pay additional co-pay for each examination and the financial intermediary may deem repeat examinations unnecessary. In these instances, the patient may be responsible for payment in full for repeat examination incurred due to inadequate bowel preparation.[1] This can be prevented by handing out patient instruction sheet along with the bowel preparation that can be used as a step by step guide before the colonoscopy. Patients should be motivated to ask questions or call doctor's office if they have any trouble or do not understand the patient instructions.

The most important factor affecting the quality of colonoscopy results is the extent of bowel cleansing. Patient tolerance of his/her colonoscopy bowel preparation- regimen affects patient compliance and henceforth his willingness to undergo repeated examinations. Patient compliance becomes a pivotal factor as it has been shown that inadequate bowel preparation reduces the quality of colonoscopy. This in turn leads to increased procedural risks and hinders the better visualization of the colonic mucosa increasing missed polyp detection rates[2,3] There are myriad of the bowel preparation agents available in the market which can make the right choice difficult. The next section describes in detail the commonly used bowel preparation agents and measures that can enhance patient compliance and acceptability of the bowel regimen prescribed to them.

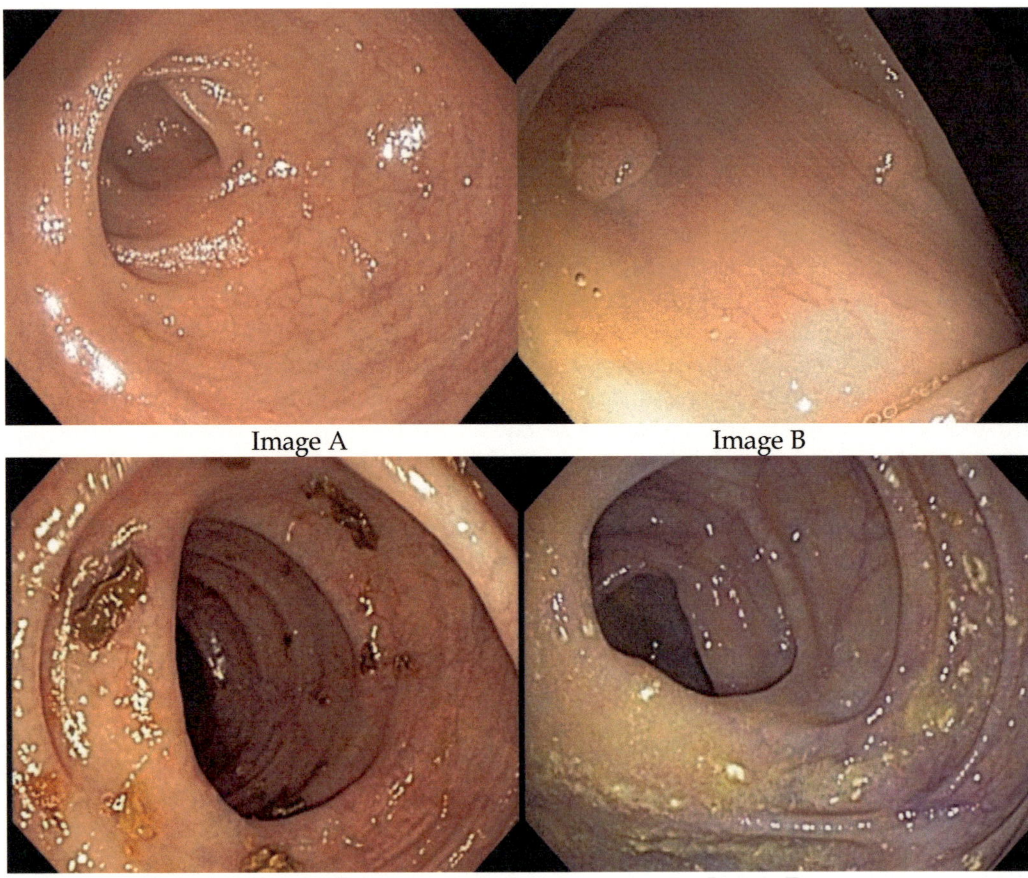

Fig. 1. Displays the images of colon with adequate and inadequate bowel preparation. Bowel preparation is excellent in images A and B allowing optimal visualization of a polyp in image B. In contrast, Images C and D have inadequate bowel preparation with solid or semisolid debris that partially obscures view of the mucosa.
(copyright permission taken from Cleveland Clinic)

2.1 Choosing the right bowel preparation agent

In general, the bowel preparation agents can be classified into one of three categories:

- Polyethylene glycol (PEG) solutions, which work as high-volume gut lavage solutions

- Osmotic agents (sodium phosphate, magnesium citrate, etc.) which draw extracellular fluid across the bowel wall and into the lumen
- Stimulants (castor oil, senna, sodium picosulfte, and bisacodyl), which work by increasing smooth muscle activity within the wall of the colon.

In current conditions, often the decision rests between using PEG or one of the osmotic agents. Stimulants are now mainly used as adjuncts to bowel preparation. Details about each agent and their pros and cons are specified below:

2.1.1 Polyethylene glycol

PEG solutions are the most commonly used bowel preparation options. They are non-absorbable and thus pass through the bowel without any net absorption and thus do not induce any substantial shifts in fluid and electrolyte levels.
Most of the commercially available PEG Preparations can be classified into the following three groups -

Standard PEG solution

Traditionally, 4 L PEG solution (CoLyte, GoLYTELY) are given the night before the colonoscopy. These are inexpensive and covered by the insurance companies. The main disadvantage is the poor palatability and large volume which causes compliance issues with 5-15% of the patients. [4,5] Large volumes are required to achieve a cleansing effect, and since this can be difficult to tolerate, nowadays split-dosing is recommended to enhance patient compliance (see patient instructions for details on split-dose standard PEG solutions).

Flavored PEG solutions

In order to decrease the salty-taste and "rotten-egg" smell from standard sulfate containing PEG solutions, attempts have been made to make sulfate free PEG solutions(SF-PEG). SF-PEG solutions in US are available in various flavors (NuLytely and TriLyte). The patient tolerance is better and it is as effective as PEG in terms of effective colonic cleansing. [6]

Low volume PEG solutions

Drinking large volume like 4 L is one of the main issues with the standard PEG solutions. Hence, several efforts have been made to reduce the volume related side effects like bloating (see section below-making bowel preparation more tolerable). Low-volume polyethylene glycol preparations such as HalfLytely and MoviPrep were developed to improve patient tolerance by reducing the amount of solution required, while maintaining efficacy by adding bisacodyl or ascorbic acid. [7-10]

Advantages of PEG solutions

- Standard PEG solutions are affordable and covered by most insurance
- Safe in patients with the electrolyte disorders
- Safe in advanced liver disease
- Can be administered safely in poorly compensated congestive heart failure or renal failure (under supervision)

Disadvantages

- Large amount of solution 4L required to achieve a cathartic effect and this affects the patient compliance terribly

- Poor salty taste in standard sulfate containing solutions affecting compliance
- Contraindicated in patients with allergies to PEG compounds, gastric outlet obstruction, high grade small bowel obstruction, significant colon obstruction, perforation, diverticulitis and hemodynamic instability
- Rarely are they associated with Mallory Weiss tear, toxic colitis, pulmonary aspiration, hypothermia, cardiac arrhythmias, and pancreatitis, SIADH [11,12]

2.1.2 Making bowel preparation more tolerable

As mentioned in previous section, drinking large volume like 4 L is one of the main issues with the PEG solutions. Several efforts have been made towards reducing the volume related side effects like bloating and hence trying to increase the patient compliance (see table 1 for list of measures that are recommended to enhance patient acceptability of PEG solutions)

There are many studies that have compared the efficacy compared to the traditional large volume PEG solutions. One such study compared full volume 4L PEG with low volume 2L PEG combined with magnesium citrate have demonstrated equal efficacy of colon cleansing but with improved overall patient tolerance.[13] Preparation like HalfLytely uses 2 L of PEG solution in combination of bisacodyl in an attempt to achieve similar efficacy.[14] Low-volume polyethylene glycol preparations such as HalfLytely and MiraLax were developed to improve patient tolerance by reducing the amount of solution required, while still maintaining efficacy by adding bisacodyl or magnesium citrate. Studies in the past had shown 2-L solutions to be as effective as 4-L solutions in terms of colon cleansing, and to be better tolerated. [13-15] though some believe that 4 L PEG treatment is sometimes better than 36 mg senna and 2 L PEG because of fewer failures.

Studies have also compared low-volume PEG + ascorbic acid with the full dose PEG and concluded that the low volume had comparable efficacy as high-volume PEG solution but had superior palatability[16] However it was noted that the cleansing results were worse if patients received the full dose PEG + Ascorbic acid the evening before the procedure compared to the split dose. The data supported the administration of PEG + Ascorbic acid as a split dose before the procedure.[17]

Studies have also compared conventional volume (4 L) of PEG-ELS with those of a low volume (2 L) in combination with pretreatment using different laxatives, such as magnesium hydroxide (milk of magnesia) and olive oil. Addition of Olive oil was found to be superior in these studies.[i8]

Another approach in increasing patient compliance by making these bowel preparation more palatable are adding flavors : PEG-electrolyte solutions are available in multiple flavors such as cherry, citrus-berry, lemon-lime, orange, and pineapple. Gatorade, Crystal Lite, and carbohydrate-electrolyte solutions have been used to improve palatability in both PEG and NaP solutions.

Combining over-the-counter (OTC) PEG-3350 laxative powder (MiraLAX) and Gatorade or Crystal Light (or other clear liquid of choice) has also been shown to improve the taste and tolerability of the preparation. MiraLAX is gaining acceptance as a bowel cleanser for colonoscopy Although beneficial and common in certain regions of the US, combining OTC PEG laxative powder with clear fluids is not an official FDA approved preparation for bowel preparation and its use is considered off-label. Studies have shown the quality of split dose Miralax bowel preparation is inferior compared to the 4L split dose Golytely for screening colonoscopies. [19,20]

Options	Comments
Using split-bowel preparation	Enhances acceptability as well as efficacy of bowel preparation. Should be standard of care for all afternoon colonoscopies and, if practical, for morning colonoscopies
Utilizing low volume or sulfate free solution	May enhance acceptability but at an added cost to patient
Chilling the solution	Enhances acceptability without impacting cost or efficacy
Adding lemon slices or sugar-free flavor enhancers (such as Crystal Light) or lemon juice	Enhances acceptability without impacting cost or efficacy. Flavors should not be red colored.
Adding metoclopramide (5 to 10 mg) orally to prevent or treat nausea	Metaclopramide can be substituted with other anti-nausea medications. Use of anti-nausea medications is optional
Adding magnesium citrate (1 bottle, about 300 mL) in patients without renal insufficiency, or bisacodyl (two to four tablets of 5 mg each), so that the volume can be less15,16	Some commercially prepared agents come prepackaged with bisacodyl or senna tablets. Shown to have equivalent efficacy as standard 4 L PEG solutions.
Stopping further ingestion of solution once the stool is watery and clear on the morning of the procedure (for patients who can clearly understand and follow bowel preparation instructions)	Shown to be beneficial in some studies. Still not widely practiced.
Giving the solution by nasogastric tube (at a rate of 1.2–1.8 L per hour) in patients with swallowing dysfunction or altered mental status	Especially relevant for hospitalized patients who have easy access to personnel to place nasogastric tube.

Table 1. Measures that can increase patient acceptability of peg solutions

The recently updated guidelines on colorectal cancer screening by the American College of Gastroenterology recommend the best practice of " split-dosing " for both PEG and sodium phosphate preparations. This is based on the data from numerous studies that have shown that split-dosing of bowel preparations (i.e., administering the first half of an agent the night before and the second half the day of colonoscopy) achieves better results than administering a single dose the day before the procedure. When all of the bowel preparation is given on the day before examination, the interval between the last dose of preparation and the performance of colonoscopy is prolonged, the probability of poor preparation increases dramatically, particularly in the cecum and ascending colon. Splitting decreases the time between the end of bowel preparation and the start of colonoscopy leading to improved efficacy. In addition, improve tolerability results from the fact that patients have to take only half the dose at a given time. Many institutions, including ours, now routinely advise split regimens for all afternoon colonoscopies. However, for morning colonoscopies, especially when patients have to travel long distances on day of colonoscopies, splitting may have some practical limitations. Since patients are advised not to drink or eat at least 2 hours before colonoscopy to prevent the risk of aspiration during sedation, patients may have to get up early AM (some time between 3 and 5 AM) to take second half of split dosing and still may have to evacuate bowel many times during travel. [21-25]

2.1.3 Sodium phoshphate (NaP)

Sodium phosphate is commonly used for bowel cleansing before colonoscopy. It is an osmotic laxative that draws water into the bowel lumen to promote colonic cleansing. Retention of water in the lumen of the colon stimulates peristalsis and bowel movements.

In December 2008, the FDA issued a black boxed warning for prescription oral sodium phosphate about the potential for acute phosphate nephropathy. Despite the boxed warning, studies suggest that oral sodium phosphate is a safe choice in properly screened patients.[26] A 2007 cohort study of 7,897 patients with normal renal function compared oral sodium phosphate and polyethylene glycol before colonoscopy. The risk of renal dysfunction was the same in both groups [27]

Advantages

- Affordable
- More tolerable to the patient
- No need for the ingestion of large volumes such as in PEG

Disadvantage

- Case reports linking NaP bowel preparation products to acute and chronic renal insufficiency were published in 2002 [28]
- Renal failure due to hyerposphatemia (acute phosphate nephropathy) has also been reported in patients with normal kidney function. [29]
- Studies have shown that older patients have a decrease in glomerular filtration rate for six months after oral sodium phosphate intake in older patients with normal baseline creatinine levels. 30

Risk factors that increase the potential for NaP related side effects include:

- chronic kidney disease,
- bowel obstruction, and
- active colitis.
- medications (e.g., diuretics, ACE inhibitors, angiotensin receptor blockers, nonsteroidal anti-inflammatory drugs)
- hypovolemia

Commercially available NaP products

Though no longer available over the counter, NaP can still be prescribed by the physicians. Visicol and Osmoprep are the two tablets forms available. NaP-based bowel preparations are easy, quick, and safe to use. Many people prefer these products because of that fact that it is a pill preparation. This gives patients the choice of what clear fluids to take it with. In clinical trials, 95% of people who took OsmoPrep said they would choose it again.[31]

However the drawback is the large amount of the tablets that need to be consumed. Visicol is a bowel purgative that contains microcrystalline cellulose (MCC) residue that impairs full visibility during a colonoscopy. Colonoscopic visualization is decreased by MCC when NaP is used alone but is improved by the addition of laxatives on the previous day.[31] Split dosing with MCC Residue Free -NaP (RF-NaP, OsmoPrep) was associated with high overall Colon Cleansing and achieved response rates of 90%, 97%, and 100% for 28, 32, and 40 tablets, respectively, compared with 86% for Visicol. In addition, RF-NaP evening-only regimen response rates were 90% (32 tablets) and 72% (28 tablets). Transient shifts in electrolyte levels were reduced, and GI adverse events were less common with lower RF-NaP dose regimens. [32]

There have been many randomized controlled trials (RCTs) comparing polyethylene glycol (PEG) with sodium phosphate (NaP). Meta-analysis comparing RCTs published between 1990 and 2008 comparing 4-L PEG with two 45 mL doses of NaP in adults undergoing elective colonoscopy showed that NaP was more likely to be completed and to result in an excellent or good quality preparation. [33] A split-dose regimen that administered the first dose of sodium phosphate on the previous evening and a second dose on the morning of the procedure (10-12 hours apart) was significantly more effective than PEG-based regimens for colorectal cleansing in preparation for colonoscopy, sigmoidoscopy or colorectal surgery. A regimen that administered both doses of oral sodium phosphate on the day prior to the procedure offered no colorectal cleansing advantage over PEG-based regimens and was significantly less effective than the split-dose NaP administration (i.e. regimen that administered one dose on the previous evening and a second dose on the morning of the procedure). Also, it has been shown that three doses (administered 10 minutes apart) of 15 mL of oral sodium phosphate solution, each diluted in 250 mL of clear fluid was associated with less vomiting than one 45 mL dose of the solution diluted in 250 mL of clear fluid .[34]

2.1.4 Magnesium citrate and oral sodium picosulfate

Oral sodium picosulfate + magnesium citrate , consisting of sodium picosulfate (a stimulant laxative) and magnesium citrate (an osmotic laxative), is approved for use in adults (CitraFleet; Picolax) and/or adolescents and children (Picolax) in Europe and Australia as a colorectal cleansing agent prior to any diagnostic procedure (e.g. colonoscopy or x-ray examination) requiring a clean bowel and/or surgery. It is dispensed in powder form (sodium picosulfate 0.01 g, magnesium oxide 3.5 g, citric acid 12.0 g per sachet), with the magnesium oxide and citric acid components forming magnesium citrate when the powder is dissolved in water. It acts locally in the colon as both a stimulant laxative, by increasing the frequency and the force of peristalsis (sodium picosulfate component), and as an osmotic laxative, by retaining fluids in the colon (magnesium citrate component), to clear the colon and rectum of fecal contents. Sodium picosulfate/magnesium citrate may be associated with a dehydrating effect, as evidenced by a reduction in bodyweight and increased hemoglobin levels; some at-risk patients may experience postural hypotension and older patients.[35]A study investigating the quality of cleansing of sodium picosulfate (Picopreparation-3™, Pharmatel Fresenius Kabi Pty Ltd, Pymble, NSW, Australia) with different administration schedules concluded the worse quality of bowel preparation was associated with the afternoon procedures and the prior history of the constipation.[36]

For countries which do not have sodium picosulfate, a reasonable alternative is magnesium citrate (1 bottle, around 300 mL) the evening before the procedure plus either bisacodyl tablets at the same time as the magnesium citrate or enema immediately before the procedure. However, literacy comparing efficacy of magnesium citrate in combination with bisacodyl or enemas and PEG or NaP solutions, is sparse.

2.2 Adjuncts to bowel preparation

2.2.1 Diet

Dietary modifications alone, such as clear liquids, are inadequate for colonoscopy but have proven benefit as an adjunct to other cleansing methods by decreasing the formation of solid residue. Clear liquids also help maintain adequate hydration during bowel preparation and are recommended with all bowel preparation regimens.

2.2.2 Stimulant laxatives

High dose senna has been used alone for bowel preparation and studies have shown comparable efficacy and better compliance. But the limiting factors were higher incidence of abdominal pain. Recently, the adjunctive use of low dose senna with PEG solutions has been demonstrated to improve the quality of bowel preparation[36] and to reduce the amount of PEG-ELS required for effective bowel preparation. [41]. This also reduces the abdominal pain reported with high dose senna. Bisacodyl (2-4 tablets of 5 mg each) and low-dose senna (36 mg, about 4 tablets of 8.6 mg Sennakot) are now commonly used as an adjunct to low-volume PEG, achieving similar results to full-volume PEG. Based on the type of study, these agents are given within 2 to 6 hours before starting of PEG solution. [37]

2.2.3 Hyperosmolar laxatives

Magnesium citrate (1 bottle, about 300 cc) alone is also commonly used as an adjunct to low volume PEG solution with equivalent efficacy to high volume PEG solutions . In contrast, the routine use of non-absorbable carbohydrates such as mannitol and lactulose is not favored for bowel preparation since the hydrogen gas produced by bacterial fermentation of the non-absorbed carbohydrates increases the risk of explosion during electrosurgical procedures. [38]

2.2.4 Antiemetic agents

Metaclopramide (5- 10 mg), a dopamine antagonist gastroprokinetic that sensitizes tissues to the action of acetylcholine,is commonly used to address the nausea or vomiting associated with bowel preparation agents. [39]

In patients who are intolerant to metaclopramide or are at high-risk for metaclopramide related side effects (such as in elderly), alternative anti-emetic agents such as promethazine (Phenergan) or ondansetron (Zofran) can be prescribed.

2.2.5 Antifoaming agent

Simethicone (3 tablets of 80 mg each, total 240 mg dose), an anti-flatulent, anti-gas agent, is prescribed by many gastroenterologists in an attempt to reduce bubbles during colonoscopy and improve the visibility. It works by reducing the surface tension of air bubbles and causing the coalescence of small bubbles into larger ones that pass more easily with belching or flatulence. [40]

2.2.6 Enemas

Enemas are sufficient for flexible sigmoidoscopies but when used alone do not permit adequate visualization of the proximal colon during colonoscopies. They are best used as adjuncts to other bowel preparation agents when patients present with poor distal colon preparation for colonoscopy. Enemas are also useful in washing out the distal segment of bowel in patients with a proximal stoma or a de-functioned distal colon. There have been studies comparing magnesium citrate with hypertonic enemas or oral bisacodyl as the bowel preparation for sigmoidoscopy over the use of hypertonic phosphate enemas alone. It was shown that there is no statistical difference between the quality of the three bowel preparations.[42] In one study inadequately prepared patients during a 19-month period were successfully cleansed of their retained fecal contents with enemas, permitting satisfactory colonoscopic examinations. [21] Thus, for the management of patients who are sub-optimally prepared for colonoscopic examination because of retained fecal material the use of colonoscopic enema proves to be effective by avoiding the need for postponement of the procedure.[43]

The common types of enema are tap water, soap suds, Fleet (NaP), Fleet-Bisacodyl and mineral oil enemas

2.2.7 Tap water enemas

500 cc to 1L tap water enemas are commonly used for bowel cleansing on the evening prior or the morning of the procedure along with the dietary restrictions and cathartics, especially for flexible sigmoidoscopies. They usually work within 10–15 minutes but may need to be repeated one or two times to thoroughly cleanse the bowel in preparation for a bowel exam or bowel surgery. In general, tap water enemas are thought to be mild enemas and may be less effective than other forms of enemas. They have fewer side effects than NaP enemas though large or repeated amounts of tap water can still lead to electrolyte imbalances as the water is absorbed through the rectum and colon. Some people differentiate between high and low enemas. A high enema is usually administered at higher pressure and with larger volume (1,000 cc), and the patient is asked to change position several times in order for the fluid to flow up into the bowel. A low enema is administered at lower pressure, using about 500 cc of fluid.

2.2.8 Soap suds enemas

Soap suds enemas are thought to be more effective than plain tap water enemas. Soaps act as surfactant and make water a more aggressive solvent. This allows the bowel content to become more liquid. Soaps are also irritant to colon and lead to increased peristalsis and evacuation of bowel content. Some soaps are safer to use than others. In general, 2 to 3 drops of hand soap are added into an enema bag filled with 2 quarts of warm filtered water.

2.2.9 NaP enemas

Sodium Biphosphate (Fleet enemas) can be used for bowel cleansing before sigmoidoscopy. However this should be avoided in elderly and in those with renal failure because of the risk of developing hyperphosphatemia and subsequent hypocalcemia. In one study, one hundred and two consecutive patients were randomized: 56 to the Fleet enema group and 46 to the Picolax group (sodium picosulfate + magnesium citrate). It was found that Fleet enemas provided a significantly superior bowel preparation with 93% being judged as adequate or better as opposed to 74% in the Picolax group. In addition Fleet enemas were associated with lesser adverse symptoms. It was thus concluded that Fleet enema is superior to Picolax in terms of bowel preparation for flexible sigmoidoscopy and the incidence of associated adverse symptoms.[44]

2.2.10 Mineral oil enemas

Mineral Oil is a lubricant laxative that works by slowing the absorption of water from the bowel which softens the stool. They are best reserved for refractory constipation. Possible side effects of mineral oil enema are:

- Bloating, diarrhea, gas, nausea, stomach cramps.
- Mineral oil enema is not recommended for use in children younger than 2 years of age. Safety and effectiveness in this age group have not been confirmed.
- Pregnancy and Breastfeeding: If the patient becomes pregnant, it is advised to discuss with their doctor the benefits and risks of using Mineral Oil Enema during pregnancy. It is unknown if Mineral Oil Enema is excreted in breast milk. Breastfeeding patients must discuss the potential side effects with their doctor.
- Patients should seek medical attention right away if any of these SEVERE side effects occur:
  - Severe allergic reactions (rash; hives; difficulty breathing; tightness in the chest; swelling of the mouth, face, lips, or tongue); dizziness.
  - Failure to have a bowel movement within 6 to 8 hours after using Mineral Oil Enema; fainting; muscle cramps or pain; rectal bleeding; swelling, pain, or irritation; weakness

2.2.11 Bisacodyl enemas

A laxative which is used for treating constipation can also be used to empty the bowel before surgery and examinations such as X-Ray procedures using Barium enema. Bisacodyl can be used as tablet, suppository or as enema. It can also be combined with NaP and other enemas. However due precautions must be taken in the following cases.

1. If the patient is allergic to Bisacodyl, aspirin or any ingredients in these products.
2. In case the patient is pregnant, Breast-feeding or plans to become pregnant.

The side effects that may be experienced during the use of Bisacodyl enema are:

- stomach cramps
- upset stomach
- diarrhea
- stomach and intestinal irritation
- faintness
- irritation or burning in the rectum (from suppositories)

2.2.12 Nasogastric tubes

Nasogastric tubes have been used to instill colonic preparations, especially for inpatients not able to drink PEG solutions or those who are unresponsive or mechanically ventilated. It can also be useful for rapid bowel cleansing

(within 2 to 3 hours) for patients with lower gastrointestinal bleeding. However, routine use of nasogastric tube solely for bowel preparation is discouraged as it can lead to severe complications, such as aspiration, in addition to trauma, during insertion. [44]

2.3 Special situations

2.3.1 Capsule endoscopy

Our practice has been to place all patients on clear liquid diet and limit the bowel preparation to patients who have recently taken or actively taking iron supplements. On the other hand, some practices routinely use oral bowel preparation for capsule endoscopy not only to clean the colon, but also to promote capsule propulsion. For hospitalized patients who are unable to take bowel preparation easily, we recommend use of nasogastric tube to deliver PEG solutions before capsule endoscopy, whenever indicated.

2.3.2 Pouchoscopy

Patients are usually prepared by taking clear liquids for 1 day before the procedure. Some practices (including ours) routinely use enemas to clear the pouch and distal small bowel before pouchoscopies. Full bowel preparation is not required for pouchoscopies.

2.3.3 Ileostomy and colostomy

Bowel preparation is not needed for scoping through the ileostomy and in-fact may be relatively contraindicated is some cases due to the risk of increasing stoma output and causing dehydration. Bowel preparation for colostomy varies by site of colostomy and practice preference. For sigmoid colostomy, many physicians chose to give full bowel preparation. It is also preferable if the patients are on clear liquids for 1 day before the procedure, especially if they have a colostomy.

2.3.4 Flexible sigmoidoscopy

Usually, enemas given within 2 hours of examination are adequate for bowel preparation for flexible sigmoidoscopy. Clear liquid diet for 1 day before procedure is optional. If patients are having diarrhea, then enemas are unnecessary. Many physicians chose not to give enemas to patients who have severe colitis, because of ongoing diarrhea and the potential for increased perforation risk.

2.3.5 Decompressive colonoscopy for megacolon

Decompressive colonoscopy is an exception when it comes to bowel preparation. Endoscopic decompression of the colon relieves acute pseudo-obstruction and megacolon in about 85% of patients but is associated with a perforation rate of about 2%. Because of the risk for colonic perforation, oral bowel preparation or enemas are avoided in these patients and decompressive colonoscopy is best done in unprepped bowel. Patients are mostly NPO in these settings.

2.3.6 Stricturing disease

In our experience, many patients with ileal or colon strictures can successfully tolerate bowel preparation (including PEG). However, their symptoms need to be watched carefully and bowel preparation should be withheld if any significant nausea, vomiting or abdomen pain develops. Patients with high-grade strictures may not tolerate oral bowel preparation and may need enemas. Bowel preparation is contraindicated in patients with suspicion of bowel obstruction.

2 weeks before colonoscopy:	**Please let your primary care physician or the prescribing physician know if you are** Taking blood thinners or antiplatelet agents such as warfarin(Coumadin), enoxaparin (Lovenox), fondaparinux (Arixtra), clopidogrel (Plavix), ticlopidine (Ticlid), anagrelide (Agrylin),cilostazol (Pletal), pentoxyphylline (trental), dipyridamole (Persantine) with aspirin (Aggrenox) Over-the-counter medications like aspirin or other anti-inflammatory medications (motrin, advil, aleve etc) might need to be stopped as well Have diabetes and take insulin. You may need to have your insulin adjusted the day before and the day of the procedure It is important to continue to take all other prescribed medications
2-5 days before the procedure:	If you tend to be constipated, maintain clear, liquid diet for two days prior to the exam. Do not take bulk-forming agents (such as Metamucil, Citrucel etc.) Do not take iron-containing preparations (such as multi-vitamins containing iron) Do not consume dairy products. Arrange for a driver to take you back home after the procedure Purchase your prescription 2 - 5 days before colonoscopy. Do not mix the solution until the before colonoscopy
Evening of the exam:	Do not add sugar or flavorings containing sugar to the solution. Refrigerating the solution, adding lemon juice or Crystal Lite and rapidly drinking 8 ounce portions (instead of sipping) may help. At 6:00 p.m. the evening before the procedure, begin drinking 8 ounces (240 ml, one cup) of the GoLYTELY every 15- 20 minutes until half of the solution is ingested. Continue drinking clear liquids until you go to bed. Do not eat solid foods for 24 hours before colonoscopy appointment. Do not take alcohol Do not take red-colored drinks, Jell-O or popsicles It is essential to drink at least 8 ounces of clear liquids (1 cup) every hour while awake to avoid dehydration. Clear liquids include: - apple or white grape juice - broth - coffee or tea (without milk or creamer) - clear carbonated beverages, such as ginger ale or lemon-lime soda - Gatorade or other sports drinks (not red) - Kool-Aid or other flavored drinks (not red) - plain Jell-O or other gelatins (not red) - popsicles (not red) - water Some people do experience nausea when drinking so much liquid, so the physician may prescribe an anti-nausea medication in case it is needed. Golytely now comes in several flavors to make it easier to drink.

Morning of the exam:	Ask your doctor if you should take any of your medicines the morning of your test. If so, take with sips of water only. If you have an afternoon appointment, begin drinking remaining GoLYTELY about 8 ounces every 10 minutes at 6:00 a.m. on the morning of the procedure, until finished at approximately 8:00 a.m. If your procedure is scheduled in early morning, you will need to get up in the night to finish the second half of GoLYTELY at least 2-3 hours before the colonoscopy appointment or complete the entire GoLYTELY in the evening before the procedure. You should drink clear liquids at least 8 ounces of clear liquids every hour (no solids, alcohol or red colored drinks) until 2 hours before colonoscopy appointment. You may take your morning medications. If the eliminations do not become clear after the gallon is finished an enema may be needed
After the exam:	The colonoscopy generally takes 30-60 minutes You must have someone else drive you back home as sedation might take some time to wear off You can resume the solid diet on the same day after the procedure.You however should continue taking more liquids. After the colonoscopy, you are encouraged to drink fluids to prevent dehydration.

2.4 Patient Instructions

Educating patients about bowel preparation instructions is critical for ensuring adequate bowel preparation and helps reduce the risk of preparation related adverse events. Patients on blood thinners, or who are diabetics, need additional instructions from their treating physicians to find the best approach in continuing or withholding some of their medications during bowel preparation.

2.4.1 General patient instruction sheet for split-dose PEG administration (with permission from Cleveland Clinic)

Follow the schedule in the table below for your bowel preparation. You may need to get to the toilet right away. You will have many bowel movements through the day. They will become very watery. The bowels are clear or clean when there is only pale yellow fluid without flecks of stool.

2.4.2 Key role of adequate hydration

One of the key concepts to emphasize to patients is the need for adequate hydration during bowel preparation. Many patients mistakenly believe that taking 4 L of polyethylene glycol obviates the need for additional hydration, since they are already ingesting such a large volume of fluid. Given that bowel preparations induce diarrhea and, in some instances, nausea and decreased oral intake, all patients taking bowel preparations are at risk of dehydration.[32] Hence, many safety issues associated with bowel preparation agents are related to dehydration and its complications.

In general, patients should be advised to consume at least 64 oz (approximately 2 L) of clear fluid on the day before the colonoscopy. According to the American Society of

Anesthesiologists, clear liquids can be safely ingested up until 2 hours before receiving anesthesia.[33] Patients should also be advised to keep drinking extra fluids after the procedure is completed to reduce the risk of dehydration and its complications

3. Conclusion

Adequate bowel preparation is essential before colonoscopy. Choosing an agent can be confusing, especially with so many agents available in the market today. Polyethylene glycol solutions are safe and effective, and are the preferred agents for cleansing the colon. Sodium phosphate can still be prescribed for patients who cannot tolerate polyethylene glycol solutions, provided they are not at risk of electrolyte or fluid imbalances. Enemas, bisacodyl, and metoclopramide are mainly used as adjuncts to polyethylene glycol but by themselves are inadequate for cleansing the entire colon. In this chapter, we have reviewed the advantages and disadvantages of available regimens, provided bowel preparation instructions for patients and emphasized the need to consider split-dose regimens as well as the need for adequate hydration before and after colonoscopy.

4. References

[1] Wexner SD, Beck DE, et al. A consensus document on bowel preparation before colonoscopy: preparationared by a task force from the American Society of Colon and Rectal Surgeons (ASCRS), the American Society for Gastrointestinal Endoscopy (ASGE), and the Society of American Gastrointestinal and Endoscopic Surgeons (SAGES). Dis Colon Rectum. 2006; 49(6):792-809

[2] Harewood GC, Sharma VK, Et al. Impact of colonoscopy preparation quality on detection of suspected colonic neoplasia. Gastrointest Endosc. 2003 ;58(1):76-9.

[3] Hendry PO, Jenkins JT, et al. The impact of poor bowel preparation on colonoscopy: a prospective single centre study of 10,571 colonoscopies. Colorectal Dis. 2007;9(8):745-8.

[4] Golub RW, Kerner BA, et al. Colonic preparations-which one? A blinded, prospective, randomized trial. Dis Colon Rectum 1995;58:594-7.

[5] Marshall JB, Pineda JJ, et al. Prospective, randomized trial comparing sodium phosphate solution with polyethylene glycol electrolyte lavage for colonoscopy preparation. Gastrointest Endosc 1993;39:631-4.

[6] DiPalma JA, Marshall JB, et al. Comparison of a new sulfate-free polyethylene glycol lavage solution versus a standard solution for colonoscopy cleansing. Gastrointest Endosc 1990;36:285-9.

[7] DiPalma JA, Wolff BG, et al. Comparison of reduced volume versus four liters sulfate-free electrolyte lavage solutions for colonoscopy colon cleansing. Am J Gastroenterol 2003; 98:2187–2191.

[8] Adams WJ, Meagher AP, et al Bisacodyl reduces the volume of polyethylene glycol solution required for bowel preparation. Dis Colon Rectum 1994; 37:229–233.

[9] Sharma VK, Steinberg EN,et al. Randomized, controlled study of pretreatment with magnesium citrate on the quality of colonoscopy preparation with polyethylene glycol electrolyte lavage solution.Gastrointest Endosc 1997; 46:541–543.

[10] Stratton S, Shelton P, et al. Feasibility of polyethylene glycol (PEG) 3350 (Miralax) for colon pre paration prior to lower endoscopic examination in healthy adults; experience in a community clinic setting. Dig Dis Sci 2011 Feb;56(2):273-5.

[11] Clark LE, DiPalma JA, et al. Safety issues regarding colonic cleansing for diagnostic and surgical procedures. Drug Saf. 2004;27:1235-42.
[12] Nelson DB, Barkun AN, et al. Technology Status evaluation report. Colonoscopy preparation, May 2001. Gastrointest Endosc. 2001; 54; 829-32.
[13] Sharma VK, Steinberg EN, et al. Randomized, controlled study of pretreatment with magnesium citrate on the quality of colonoscopy preparation with polyethylene glycol electrolyte lavage solution. Gastrointest Endosc.1997;46:541-3.
[14] Adams WJ, Meagher AP, et al. Bisacodyl reduces the volume of PEG solution required for bowel preparation. Dis Colon Rectum. 1994;27:229-33.
[15] Haapamäki MM, Lindström M, et al. Low-volume bowel preparation is inferior to standard 4 1 polyethylene glycol. Surg Endosc. 2011 Mar;25(3):897-901.
[16] Coporaal S, KleibeukerJH, et al. Low-volume PEG plus ascorbic acid versus high-volume PEG as bowel preparation for colonoscopy. Scand J Gastroenterology 2010 Nov; 45(11): 1380-6.
[17] Marmo R, Rotondano G, et al. Effective bowel cleansing before colonoscopy: a randomized study of split-dosage versus non-split dosage regimens of high-volume versus low-volume polyethylene glycol solutions. Gastrointest Endosc. 2010 Aug;72(2):313-20.
[18] Abut E, Guveli H, et al. Administration of olive oil followed by a low volume of polyethylene glycol-electrolyte lavage solution improves patient satisfaction with right-side colonic cleansing over administration of the conventional volume of polyethylene glycol-electrolyte lavage solution for colonoscopy preparation. Gastrointest Endosc. 2009;70(3):515-21.
[19] Hjelkrem M, Stengel J, et al. MiraLAX Is Not as Effective as GoLytely in Bowel Cleansing Before Screening Colonoscopies. 2011;9(4):326-332.e1.
[20] Enestyedt BK, Fennerty MB, et al. Randomised clinical trial: MiraLAX vs. Golytely - a controlled study of efficacy and patient tolerability in bowel preparation for colonoscopy. 2011;33(1):33-40.
[21] Rex DK, Johnson DA, et al. American College of Gastroenterology Guidelines for Colorectal Cancer Screening 2008. Am J Gastroenterol 2009;104:739–750.
[22] Rex DK, Imperiale TF, et al. Impact of bowel preparation on efficiency and cost of colonoscopy. Am J Gastroenterol 2002; 97:1696–1700.
[23] El Sayed AM, Kanafani ZA, et al. A randomized single-blind trial of whole vs. split-dose polyethylene glycol-electrolyte solution for colonoscopy preparation. Gastrointest Endosc 2003;58:36–40.
[24] 24. Rostom A, Jolicoeur E, et al. A randomized prospective trial comparing different regimens of oral sodium phosphate and polyethylene glycol-based lavage solution in the preparation of patients for colonoscopy. Gastrointest Endosc 2006;64:544–552.
[25] 25. Park JS, Sohn CI, et al. Quality and effect of single dose vs. split dose of polyethylene glycol bowel preparation for early-morning colonoscopy. Endoscopy. 2007 Jul;39(7):616-9
[26] 26. Singal AK, Rosman AS, et al. The renal safety of bowel preparations for colonoscopy: a comparative study of oral sodium phosphate solution and polyethylene glycol. Aliment Pharmacol Ther. 2008;27(1):41–47.
[27] Russmann S, Lamerato L, et al. Risk of impaired renal function after colonoscopy: a cohort study in patients receiving either oral sodium phosphate or polyethylene glycol. Am J Gastroenterol. 2007;102(12):2655–2663.

[28] Markowitz GS, Stokes MB, et al. Acute phosphate nephropathy following oral sodium phosphate bowel purgative: an underrecognized cause of chronic renal failure. J Am Soc Nephrol. 2005;16(11):3389–3396.
[29] Hookey LC, Depew WT, et al. The safety profile of Oral sodium phosphate for colon cleansing before colonoscopy in adults. Gastrointestinal Endos. 2002;56:895-902.
[30] Rex DK, Schwartz H, et al. Safety and colon-cleansing efficacy of a new residue-free formulation of sodium phosphate tablets. Am J Gastroenterol. 2006;101:2594-2604
[31] Aihara H, Saito S, et al. Comparison of two sodium phosphate tablet-based regimens and a polyethylene glycol regimen for colon cleansing prior to colonoscopy: a randomized prospective pilot study. Int J Colorectal Dis. 2009 Sep;24(9):1023-30.
[32] Wruble L, Demicco M, et al. Residue-free sodium phosphate tablets (OsmoPrep) versus Visicol for colon cleansing Gastrointest Endosc. 2007 Apr;65(4):660-70.
[33] Juluri R, Eckert G, et al. Meta-analysis: randomized controlled trials of 4-L polyethylene glycol and sodium phosphate solution as bowel preparation for colonoscopy. Alimentary Pharmacol Ther. 2010 Jul;32(2):171-81.
[34] 34. Curran MP, Plosker GL, et al. Oral sodium phosphate solution: a review of its use as a colorectal cleanser. Drugs. 2004;64(15):1697-714.
[35] Hoy SM, Scott LJ, et al. Sodium picosulfate/magnesium citrate: a review of its use as a colorectal cleanser. Drugs. 2009;69(1):123-36
[36] Varughese S, Kumar AR, et al. Morning-only one-gallon polyethylene glycol improves bowel cleansing for afternoon colonoscopies: a randomized endoscopist-blinded prospective study. Am J Gastroenetrology 2010 Nov;105(11):2368-74.
[37] Ziegenhagen DJ, Zehnter E, et al. Addition of Senna improves colonoscopy preparation with lavage: a prospective randomized trial. Gastrointest Endosc 1991;37(5):547-9.
[38] Bigard MA, Gaucher P, Lassalle C. Fatal colonic explosion during colonoscopic polypectomy. Gastroenterology 1979; 77:1307–1310.
[39] Rhodes JB, Engstrom J, Stone KF. Metoclopramide reduces the distress associated with colon cleansing by an oral electrolyte overload. Gastrointest Endosc 1978; 24:162–163.
[40] Wu L, Cao Y, Liao C, Huang J, Gao F.Systematic review and meta-analysis of randomized controlled trials of Simethicone for gastrointestinal endoscopic visibility. Scand J Gastroenterol. 2011;46(2):227-35.
[41] Iida Y, Miura S, et al. Bowel preparation for the total colonoscopy by 2000 ml of balanced lavage solution (GoLytely) and sennoside. Gastroenterol Jpn 1992; 27(6):728-33.
[42] Fincher RK, Osgard EM, et al. Comparison of bowel preparations for flexible sigmoidoscopy: oral magnesium citrate combined with oral bisacodyl, one hypertonic phosphate enema, or two hypertonic phosphate enemas. Am J Gastroenterol. 1999;94(8):2122-7.
[43] Sohn N, Weinstein MA, et al.Management of the poorly preparationared colonoscopy patient: colonoscopic colon enemas as a preparation for colonoscopy. 2008;51(4):462-6.
[44] P.J Drew, M. Hughes, et al. The optimal bowel preparation for flexible sigmoidoscopy. European Journal of surgical oncology, 1997; 23:315–316.

4

Monitoring During Colonoscopy

Rosalinda S. Hulse
Jordan Hospital, Plymouth, MA
USA

1. Introduction

Many individuals are still hesitant to undergo colonoscopy despite numerous advertisements and campaigns about it. A few years back, a famous TV personality named Katie Kouric, had her colonoscopy broadcasted through live television because she wanted the public to see that there's nothing scary or frightening about the procedure. Her husband died of colon cancer at a young age. Had he had a colonoscopy (Fig. 1), his cancer would have been diagnosed and treated early which could have saved or prolonged his life.

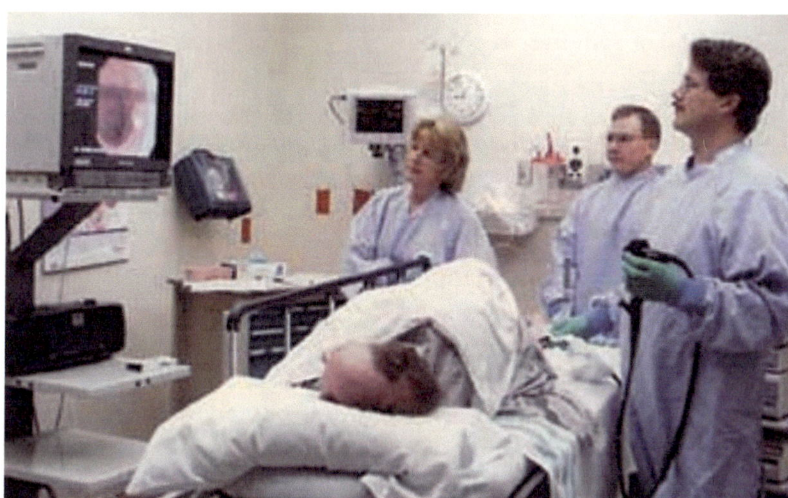

Fig. 1. Colonoscopy.

The test remains an uncomfortable, frightening, and embarrassing and anxiety producing situation, especially for people undergoing it for the first time, which can then lead to delays in screening and treatment. Though endoscopic procedures can be performed and tolerated without sedation, studies have shown that "16% to 56% of such procedures are terminated because of pain".[22] The goal of colonoscopy is to reach the cecum (the beginning of the large intestine). The scope is less likely to reach that destination, as it navigates the long and tortuous colon, without adequate sedation. Figure 2 shows the colon or large intestine and its location in the abdomen.

Many countries around the world commonly perform colonoscopy without sedation. [12] In Japan, though endoscopic procedures are routinely carried out without sedation, many Japanese are now choosing this to ease the discomfort.[32] Only 2%-7% would prefer this option in the United States.[29]

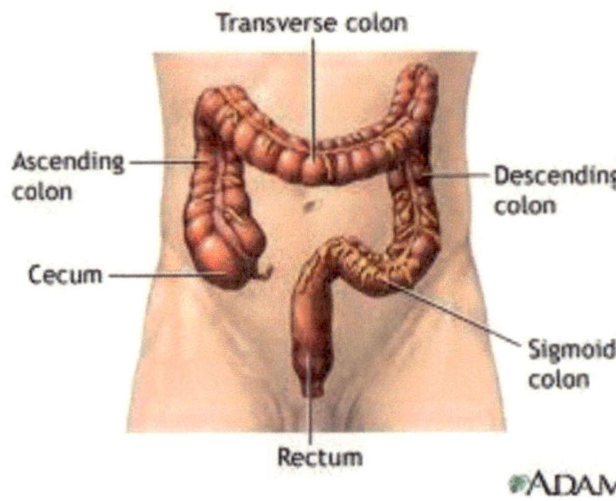

Fig. 2. The colon or large intestine

The challenge and goal of sedation in colonoscopy is to effectively facilitate the procedure while relieving anxiety, pain or discomfort, providing amnesia, and preserving cardiopulmonary function of the individual, with minimal cognitive impairment post procedure. This may delay the individual's discharge from the hospital. Sedation is now the standard of practice for endoscopic procedures in the U.S. and in many other countries. It is necessary to complete the procedure with ease and comfort.[26,19,21,23,9,32,31,38] Currently used medications are: benzodiazepines (e.g., midazolam, diazepam), opioids (e.g., meperidine, sublimaze), and propofol. Ketamine and inhaled anesthetics (e.g. nitrous oxide) are rarely used because of their side effects and uneasiness of administration.[23,22] These drugs are used alone or in combination with another drug. Comparison studies have been done to determine which combination of drugs are better in minimizing cognitive impairment post procedure, but none have been found to be better than the other.[21] The ideal amount of sedation for a patient undergoing colonoscopy has also not been established despite the many different techniques, medications and combinations thereof attempted.

This chapter will discuss the different types of moderate sedation given, who will be administering it, and how individuals are monitored during the procedure. The goal is to inform the public of the different methods of making one comfortable during colonoscopy. Emphasis will be given to the fact that this procedure is short and safe, and usually does not require administration of heavy-duty anesthetics or sedatives. Monitoring is done frequently with particular attention to the airway, breathing (using pulse oximetry and capnography) and circulation i.e., heart rate and blood pressure. Knowledge of the availability of these medications will make the individual feel confident that he or she will be comfortable and cared for during his or her colonoscopy.

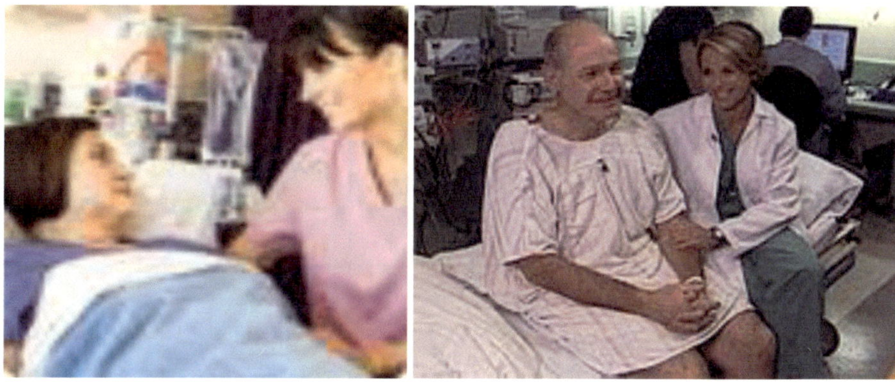

Fig. 3. Confidence and satisfaction in colonoscopic procedures

2. Safety and efficacy of currently used sedation drugs for colonoscopy

Sedation is defined as the calming of mental excitement or abatement of physiologic functions with the administration of a drug,[31] i.e. a drug-induced depression of the individual's level of consciousness.[4] As mentioned earlier, sedation is recommended in most endoscopic procedures to facilitate completion of the procedure, which in this case, would be colonoscopy.

Four levels characterize sedation: minimal or light (anxiolysis) sedation, moderate sedation (formerly known as conscious sedation), deep sedation, and general anesthesia.[2] The most commonly used in colonoscopy is moderate sedation, where the patient continues to respond purposefully to verbal commands, with or without light touch stimulation. He is spontaneously breathing on his own and may be supported with minimal amounts of oxygen via a nasal cannula or sometimes a mask may be necessary. In deeply sedated states, patients may not be roused easily, and respond only after repeated or painful stimuli. They may also not have spontaneous respirations (breathing on their own) requiring assistance to maintain a patent airway. General anesthesia is normally reserved for surgical procedures wherein patients do not respond to any form of stimulation, are completely immobile and support of his or her cardiovascular functioning is required.[4] Table 1 shows summary of the various levels of sedation and analgesia. Adapted from the American Society of Anesthesiologists Standards and Guidelines (2009).[2]

Moderate anesthesia care (MAC) and/or moderate level of sedation (also formerly known as conscious sedation) is usually employed during colonoscopy. It allows for better patient cooperation and a quicker or shorter recovery time.[26] Individuals certified to administer the drugs and monitor the patient's response(s), such as a gastroenterologist, a registered nurse, a certified registered nurse anesthetist, or an anesthesiologist, can safely administer this.[32] However, there are some differences between MAC and moderate sedation. During moderate sedation, a physician personally administers or supervises a nurse to administer the sedative and/or analgesic drug. These individuals are qualified and certified to administer the sedation drugs maintaining the level of sedation to a "moderate" or lesser degree. They continually monitor and assess the effects of these drugs and level of sedation the patient is in throughout the duration of the procedure, are competent to recognize changes especially when the individual goes into a deeper level than originally intended and, are able to manage the consequences and adjust additional doses of the medication to maintain the desired level of consciousness.

	Minimal or Light Sedation (Anxiolysis)	Moderate Sedation or Analgesia (Conscious Sedation)	Deep Sedation or Analgesia	General Anesthesia
Responsiveness	Normal response to verbal stimuli	Purposeful response to verbal or tactile stimuli	Purposeful response following repeated or painful stimuli	Unarousable even with repeated or painful stimuli
Airway	Unaffected	No intervention required	Intervention may be required	Intervention is often required
Spontaneous Ventilation	Unaffected	Adequate	Maybe inadequate or compromised	Frequently inadequate and is compromised
Cardiovascular Function	Unaffected	Usually maintained	Usually maintained	Maybe impaired

Table 1. Summary of the various levels of sedation and analgesia. Adapted from the American Society of Anesthesiologists, Standards and Guidelines, 2009. [2]

In moderate sedation, the provider assigned to observing and monitoring the patient as well as administering the sedation medications has other responsibilities and tasks that are interruptible and of short duration. The reverse is true for moderate anesthesia care or MAC, where the provider (usually an anesthesiologist or nurse anesthetist) is solely dedicated to the observation and monitoring of the patient and does not have any other procedure-related responsibilities. He must be prepared to convert to general anesthesia when the patient's cardiorespiratory status is compromised. It is an essential component of his initial assessment to evaluate the patient's actual or anticipated physiological problem that may compromise his cardiorespiratory status during the scheduled procedure. His ability to rescue a patient whose airway is compromised is a prerequisite to his ability to provide moderate anesthesia care. The administration of hypnotics, sedatives and analgesics, as well as other drugs commonly used for the induction and maintenance of general anesthesia is often, but not always, a part of monitored anesthesia care.[4]

Since sedation is a continuum, it is impossible to predict how an individual will respond to the drugs. Some patients may require only small amounts of sedation, but MAC is often indicated because even small doses of these medications could precipitate adverse physiologic responses that would require acute clinical interventions and resuscitation. If a patient's health status or condition, or medical/surgical history is likely to require sedation to a deeper level or even to a momentary period of general anesthesia, then MAC is the preferred method. Due to the strong possibility that a deep or deeper level of sedation may transition to general anesthesia, the skills and expertise of an anesthesia provider (e.g.

anesthesiologist or certified registered nurse anesthetist, CRNA) are essential to manage the effects of general anesthesia as well as the patient's quick return to a lesser state of sedation. MAC also includes post-procedure responsibilities such as ensuring return to full consciousness, complete relief of pain, management of side effects or any adverse physiologic responses from the drugs administered during the procedure, as well as the diagnosis and treatment of some co-existing medical problems.[2]

Since individuals vary in their responses to the sedation medication, and may be in different levels of sedation as well, while undergoing the same procedure, or may require different levels to complete the procedure; it is imperative that clinicians administering the sedatives/analgesics and monitoring their effects have the necessary skills and knowledge in recognizing complications associated with sedation/analgesia, and be able to rescue or resuscitate the individual whose sedation status is deeper than originally intended.[4,37] They must have also undergone a course or class and be certified in cardiopulmonary resuscitation (CPR) as well as in Advanced Cardiac Life Support (ACLS).[20,16,37,3] In patients with significantly sedation-related risk factors, i.e., severe obstructive pulmonary disease, sleep apnea, potentially difficult airway, congestive heart failure, and coronary artery disease, the presence of an anesthesiologist is highly recommended. It is also recommended for patients who may require a deeper level of sedation to achieve adequate procedure result, such as individuals who are on high doses of psychotropic medications, benzodiazepines, alcohol, and narcotics.[4,22,3]

Class	**Description**
ASA I	A normal healthy patient
ASA II	Patient has mild systemic disease which does not interfere with daily activities, such as high blood pressure that is under control
ASA III	Patient has a moderate or severe systemic disease that does not inhibit or limit daily activities such as diabetes with some systemic complications
ASA IV	Patient has a severe systemic disease that is a constant threat to life such as end-stage renal or liver failure, or congestive heart failure
ASA V	The patient is moribund and is not expected to survive within 24 hours, with or without the procedure
ASA VI	The patient is declared brain-dead and his or her organs are being removed for donation purposes.
E	In addition to indicating the ASA status, a patient undergoing an emergency procedure is indicated by the suffix "E."

Table 2. Patient status classification according to the American Society of Anesthesiologists (ASA)

Many studies have been performed regarding administration of these drugs during colonoscopy and were found to provide safe and effective sedation during the procedure, especially when titrated in small incremental doses. Though safe and effective, these drugs do carry potential problems or concerns that include cardiopulmonary events, such as hypotension, airway obstruction, hypoxia/hypoxemia, aspiration, apnea, arrhythmia, vasovagal episodes, and though uncommon, serious morbidity and death can also occur.[24,15,16] A review of data from the American Society for Gastrointestinal Endoscopy's (ASGE) computer-based management system of 21,000 GI endoscopies in 1988 using Versed (Midazolam) and Valium (Diazepam) revealed the following: Overall complication rate was 13.5 events per 1000 procedures and serious cardiopulmonary events were 5.4 per 1000. Death occurred in 0.3 per 1000.[5] Another study evaluating the safety of the combination of meperidine (Demerol) with either midazolam (Versed) or diazepam (Valium) revealed no deaths.6 Results from two other studies showed a considerably lower incidence of cardiopulmonary complications using propofol as compared with the use of benzodiazepines during routine endoscopic procedure.[38,25,28] Because of these potential complications, endoscopy suites are equipped with the tools necessary to rescue the patient. These include: a suction machine, oxygen outlet or tank, a code cart with a defibrillator, a bag-valve mask, oral and nasal airways, a nasogastric tube, materials for respiratory intubation, and drugs required for cardiorespiratory resuscitation.[20]

3. Economics of sedation in endoscopy

In the past, gastroenterologists have routinely administered the sedating agents to their patients as part of the colonoscopy service. However, in recent years, many endoscopists are employing the services of an anesthesiologist or a certified registered nurse anesthetist (CRNA) to administer the sedation. The influencing factors being, the increased use of propofol during this procedure, effective marketing by anesthesiologists, and by a decrease in reimbursements by insurers.[4,35]

The approach of individual countries towards administration of sedatives and analgesics during colonoscopy varies widely due to differences in health insurance reimbursements and budget restraints.[41,22] In the United States, Medicare reimbursements for use of an anesthesiologist during colonoscopy are not uniform across the nation. Some health insurers also question the separate billing of anesthesia service when generally; reimbursement fee for the colonoscopy includes administration of sedation under the supervision of the gastroenterologist.[1]

Ideally, an anesthesiologist is present in all cases of colonoscopy to optimize sedation and analgesia. However, his presence during this short procedure for individuals who are at average-risk for developing sedation-related complications is debatable and not cost-effective.[1] Normally, these patients are able to maintain their airway with minimal or no support so that the skills of an anesthesiologist is not necessary. Many studies have been done exploring the use of a registered nurse administering propofol and have found safety levels equivalent to those administered with benzodiazepines and narcotics.[32,33,30,36]

4. Colonoscopy without sedation

In some instances, few selected patients opt to undergo their colonoscopy without sedation. In the US, a survey found that only 2% to 7% of individuals were willing to do their colonoscopies without sedation.29 Review of literature found no randomized control trials done to compare sedation versus no sedation during colonoscopy. Many argue that they want to watch the procedure and are fascinated by what's inside the human body. Some are unable to find an available designated driver and are unwilling to reschedule their appointment. Still some have stated that they have a lot of commitments and things to do that they cannot afford to skip a day to rest at home. In some rare instances, the individual went straight to work after his procedure. The type and level of monitoring should be tailored to each individual in these cases. Often, the individual is advised to bring a designated driver, in case he changes his mind and decides to receive sedation. Men, patients who are generally healthy and have no history of abdominal pain, individuals who are not anxious, and older patients may be better able to tolerate the colonoscopy without sedation. In situations like this, a smaller diameter endoscope (pediatric scope) is used and is better tolerated.

5. Preprocedure assessment and monitoring

A few weeks prior to the scheduled colonoscopy, the patient usually pays his endoscopist a visit to review his general state of health, medical and surgical histories, allergies, and regularly taken medications. Special instructions will be given to diabetics with regards to intake of their medications as well as diet. The appropriate bowel cleansing prep will be reviewed and instructions provided. The patient will also be informed that he will be receiving sedating medications to make the procedure more comfortable and tolerable. He is then advised to arrange for someone to drive him home because he will not be allowed to drive home, take the bus or taxi after the procedure due to the residual effects of the sedative; emphasizing the fact that these side effects do alter his reflexes and cognitive functioning. This usually wears off in about four to six hours; and, even after this time, the individual may still feel very tired and sleepy. Patients are discharged home and advised to take the day off and rest. They are normally allowed to eat light, non-spicy, and easily digestible foods to avoid nausea and vomiting which is often a side effect of sedatives and opioids.

The use of combination regimen as well as patient characteristics influence the safety and choice of sedative regimens for this procedure. Therefore, general data is collected from every patient, recorded in his medical record and reviewed by both the endoscopist and the personnel providing the sedating medication (s), shortly before the colonoscopy is performed. These include: name, age (determined by date-of-birth), sex, general condition of health (as outlined in the ASA classification, Table 2), daily medications taken, allergies, medical and surgical histories, adverse reactions to sedatives and anesthetics, and problems (if any) post procedure or surgery. The following historical events should also be obtained from the patient: any significant abnormalities of major organ or organ systems, snoring or sleep apnea (using CPAP or BiPap), time and type of last meal taken, use of illicit drugs, and alcohol and tobacco use. Regarding the "time and type of last meal taken," there are no absolute or ultimate guidelines regarding the stopping of oral intake prior to administration of sedatives. There are no supporting data showing a direct relationship between fasting time and risk of aspiration into the lungs. The ASA guidelines recommend that patients not have clear liquids two hours before the procedure and a light meal six hours before administration of any sedating medication. This would allow sufficient time for the stomach to adequately empty.[4] According to the American College of Emergency Physicians, "recent food intake is not contraindicated for administering procedural sedation and analgesia, but should be considered in choosing the timing and target of sedation".[8]

Physical examination of the individual is obtained and recorded. These include, initial vital signs (temperature, heart rate, blood pressure, respiratory rate, and oxygen saturation), level of consciousness, examination of heart and lungs, and airway anatomy (using the Mallampati classification, Figure 4). The last one is important in situations where the individual may need resuscitative assistance such as: 1) individuals with a history of snoring, stridor, or sleep apnea and is using a CPAP or BiPAP machine, 2) neck abnormalities involving the neck and facial features (e.g. obese persons), short neck, limited neck extension, neck mass, cervical spine disease or trauma to the neck, tracheal deviation, advanced rheumatoid arthritis, decreased hyoid-mental distance (<3cm in adults), 3) abnormalities of the mouth such as protruding incisors, small opening (<3cm n adults), high arched palate, hypertrophy of the tonsils, nonvisible uvula (see class 4 of the Mallampati classification, Figure 4), edentulous, loose or capped teeth, macroglossia, 4) history of problems with sedation and anesthetics, 5) dysmorphic facial features such as trisomy and Pierre-Robin syndrome, and 6) jaw abnormalities such as trismus, significant malocclusion, micrognathia, and retrognathia. The ASA Task Force guideline states "that the presence of one or more sedation-related risk factors coupled with the potential for deep sedation will increase the likelihood of adverse sedation-related events." Consultation with someone trained in managing these complex situations, usually an anesthesiologist or a certified registered nurse anesthetist should be considered.[4] The presence of an anesthesiologist is also highly recommended for the following situations:

- Significantly compromised individuals such as those with congestive heart failure, coronary artery disease, and severe obstructive pulmonary disease (COPD) on continuous oxygen therapy or using CPAP or BiPAP machines
- Individuals with difficult airways (such as those described above)
- Extremely obese individuals
- ASA status classification of Class III, IV, and V
- Increased risk of pulmonary aspiration
- The individual is pregnant
- If it appears that sedation (even with small doses) will make the patient unresponsive and airway will be compromised
- General anesthesia is necessary to complete the procedure while maintaining patient safety and comfort
- Unavailability of a trained practitioner to administer moderate sedation
- Anticipated intolerance of standard sedation drugs (e.g. alcohol or substance abuse)
- Adverse reactions to sedatives
- Inadequate response to moderate sedation

A Modified Aldrete score is also assigned (see post procedure monitoring). An intravenous access is established because sedation drugs are normally given intravenously. Fluids may or may not be routinely given depending on the institution's procedural policies and regulations. For female patients, it is necessary to mention the possibility of being pregnant or is pregnant. If in doubt, a pregnancy test may be performed. Lactating mothers should also mention if they are breastfeeding as most of the medication is excreted in breast milk.

Shortly before the procedure starts, the provider of the sedating medications will discuss with the patient the type of sedating medications to be given; its benefits, risks and complications, limitations and other alternatives. The endoscopist will also review the procedure with the patient. He will then sign the consent form allowing the endoscopist to perform the procedure and to be given sedating medications (if agreeing to sedation). The anticipated level of sedation should be congruent with the expected level of sedation by the individual as much as possible. The endoscopist will also review the colonoscopy procedure, the benefits, risks and complications to patients who are not receiving sedation. Preparation is the same as for sedation in the event that an emergency arises or the patient requests medication during the procedure.

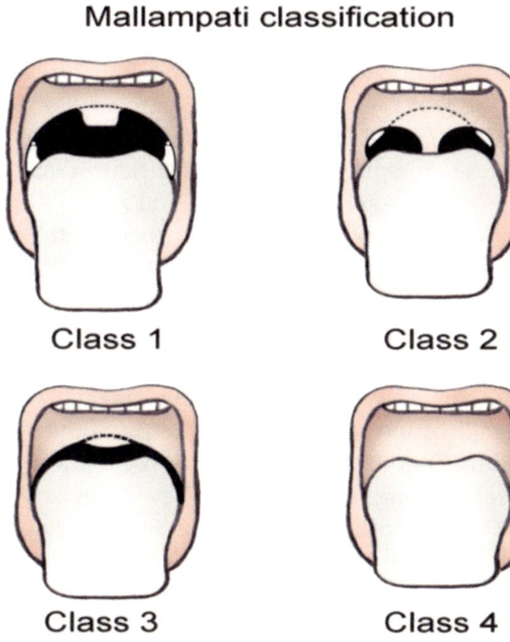

Fig. 4. Mallampati classification of airway management.

6. Sedation and monitoring during colonoscopy

According to the recommendations outlined by The Joint Commission and the Association of Anesthesiologists, hospital-based endoscopy suites consists of the following personnel: a physician endoscopist, an assisting nurse, and an additional nurse solely administering sedatives and monitoring the patient.[14] However, with the advent and increased use of propofol, there has been a demand for the presence of an anesthesiologist or certified registered nurse anesthesiologist. This is partly due to the widespread perception that the drug carries major complication risks and statements emphasized by the information on the package insert of the drug itself, recommending that only personnel trained in the administration of general anesthesia administer this drug. The ASA guidelines also outlined numerous precautions regarding the administration of propofol thereby, increasing fears of non-anesthetists. It is also the perception that administration of benzodiazepines and opiates only induce moderate level of sedation and that propofol brings the patient into a deep level sedation.[20] Several studies though have proved that propofol can be safely administered by non-anesthesiologists.[11,32,15,29]

Only 7.7% of gastroenterologists in the US administer propofol themselves without the assistance or presence of an anesthesiologist or nurse anesthetist (CRNA), and 68% have expressed interest in incorporating it in their practice given proper training and adequately trained staff.9 The reason for the reluctancy among endoscopists to administer propofol themselves, are medico legal implications of the off-label use of propofol, the potential risks and complications, local institutional policy, and state regulatory restrictions.[4] Hence, propofol is usually administered by an anesthesiologist (or by a certified registered nurse anesthetist [CRNA]) which is often not cost-effective in ambulatory gastrointestinal (GI) suites .[12] In some countries, like Switzerland, 34% of gastroenterologists polled administer propofol themselves.[15]
During the procedure, the patient is hooked up to a monitor that measures and displays the heart rate, blood pressure, and oxygen saturation (Figure 5) and in some cases, carbon dioxide levels (capnography). Some have also used transcutaneous carbon dioxide measurement or bispectral index monitoring (BIS). The latter is a quantitative assessment of cortical activity that has been used to monitor sedation and adjust sedation levels (Kissin, I., 2000). These are monitored by a licensed personnel (usually the person providing the sedation) every 3-5minutes during the procedure and with each incremental dose of the sedative. Monitoring may detect changes in the individual's blood pressure, heart rate, cardiac electrical activity, ventilatory, and neurologic status that might signal a clinically significant compromise of the patient's health status or that the patient has progressed to a deeper level of sedation than originally intended. Oxygen is usually given as an adjunct via a nasal cannula or mask as all of the sedation agents depress the respiratory system. The ASA guidelines recommend that patients receiving sedation medications receive continuous electrocardiogram (ECG) monitoring, especially if they have significant cardiovascular disease or arrhythmias.[20] Parameters outlined in the Modified Aldrete scoring system, which includes the above mentioned items plus activity and consciousness are also monitored and recorded.

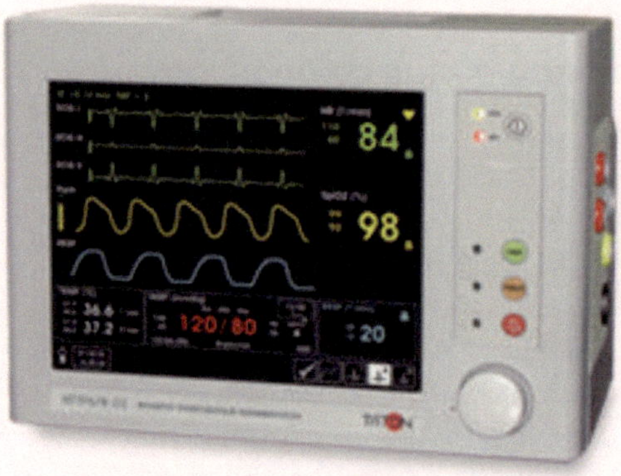

Fig. 5. Sample of monitoring equipment used

In most institutions, an intravenous access is started and IV fluids are given prior and during the procedure. This helps hydrate the patient, provide an avenue for the administration of sedating drugs, and as a rescue means should the patient become hypotensive (ASGE, 2008). Should the patient's condition get compromised or deteriorate at any given time during the procedure, the colonoscopy is halted and resuscitative measures are instituted. He may need to be transferred to the Critical Care Unit or the Emergency Department for further management.

6.1 Post procedure monitoring

Upon completion of the colonoscopy, the patient is kept in the room and monitored for a few more minutes until he is rousable and able to maintain his airway independently. Shortly thereafter, he is disconnected from all the monitoring equipment and brought to the recovery or discharge area to allow the effects of the sedatives to wear off. Here, the same parameters monitored during the procedure are monitored and recorded every 10-15 minutes for about half-an-hour to an hour, without the continuous cardiac monitoring (ECG) (unless warranted) and the carbon dioxide monitoring, until the patient is at or close to his or her baseline cognitive functioning level as possible, and is ready for discharge to home. Blood sugar levels of diabetics will also be checked and intervention given as necessary.

At this time, the endoscopist will come to discuss his findings during the procedure, any interventions done (i.e. biopsies taken), and discharge and follow-up instructions will be given. The patient's designated driver is encouraged to be present because he (the patient) may not remember what the endoscopist has said as a result of the amnesic properties of the sedatives, especially with benzodiazepines (not so with propofol), unless the patient requests otherwise. The patient is discharged when he or she has met discharge criteria as outlined by the Modified Aldrete or Aldrete and Kroulik scoring system (Tables 3 and 3.a) or whichever discharge scoring system the institution is using and has returned to his baseline (or close to it) level of cognitive and physiological functioning as possible.

Ideally, the recovery or discharge area should allow rapid recovery of the sedated individual, with minimal or without residual physiologic, cognitive or psychomotor impairments. Several discharge criteria have been formulated to facilitate and guide clinicians to objectively asses the clinical status of the sedated patient and be able to discharge him home. The most commonly used is the Modified Aldrete or Aldrete and Kroulik scoring systems (Table 3 and 3.a).[39] The preferred method is the Modified Aldrete scoring system as most institutions do not use arterial pressure monitoring for endoscopy procedures, especially in an outpatient setting. This scoring is also used pre-, inta and post procedure. During the procedure, if the patient is maintained at the moderate sedation level, his score should be a 9 or a 10 or whatever his baseline score was at the start. Over sedation is defined by a score of less than 9 and corrective action should be initiated. All post sedation patients should have their vital signs back to within 10% of their baseline score or be admitted to the hospital for further evaluation especially if corrective/resuscitative actions have failed to improve his score or condition.

Post anesthesia discharge scoring system (PADSS) has been developed for post-anesthesia care units in Canada. This allows the health care providers to monitor the patient's readiness to be discharged home. The average length of time the sedated patient stays in the discharge or recovery area is half-an-hour to an-hour depending on the kind and amount of sedation drugs received during the procedure. Patients who receive propofol generally recover quicker and are discharged home in a much shorter time than those who receive benzodiazepines or in combination thereof.[20] Prompt and safe discharge of the patients reduces the amount of time they stay in the discharge area and contributes to cost reduction and unit efficiency.[7]

Modified Aldrete Scoring		
Criteria	**Ability**	**Score**
Activity	Ability to move voluntarily or on command:	
	Four extremities	2
	Two extremities	1
	No movement	0
Respiration	Able to cough and breathe deeply freely	2
	Dyspnea, shallow or limited breathing	1
	Apnea	0
Circulation	Blood pressure within 20mm Hg of pre-sedation level	2
	Blood pressure within 20-50mm Hg of pre-sedation level	1
	Blood pressure + 50mm Hg of pre-sedation level	0
Consciousness	Fully awake	2
	Arousable on calling	1
	Not responding	0
O2 Saturation	Able to maintain O2 saturation >92% on room air	2
	Needs O2 to maintain O2 saturation >90%	1
	O2 saturation is <90% even with O2 supplementation	0

Table 3. Modified Aldrete Scoring System

Assessment Item	**Condition**	**Grade**
Muscle Activity	Moves 4 extremities	2
	Moves 2 extremities	1
	Moves 0 extremities	0
Breathing	Deep, Cough	2
	Limited, Dyspnea	1
	Apnea	0
Consciousness	Fully awake	2
	Awakens when called	1
	Does not respond to call	0
Circulation (AP)*	+ of 20% of pre-anesthesia level	2
	+ 20% to 49% of pre-anesthesia level	1
	+ 50% of pre-anesthesia level	0
SpO2**	Maintains SpO2 >92% in ambient air	2
	Maintains SpO2 > 90% with O2	1
	Maintains SpO2 <90% with O2	0

*AP = arterial pressure
** = peripheral oxygen saturation

Table 3a. Aldrete and Kroulik Index

7. Commonly used sedation agents

Colonoscopy procedures are usually done under moderate level of sedation or moderate anesthesia care (MAC). To achieve this, general practice guidelines call for the careful titration of the chosen sedative using incremental doses. The most commonly used agents are benzodiazepines, alone or in combination with an analgesic, and propofol, alone or also in combination with another agent.[21],[26],[22] The choice of sedating agent is largely dependent on the provider based on what he thinks and feels is the best in maximizing patient comfort at the same time, minimizing risks and complications. A US survey noted that over 85% of endoscopists use or prefer to use midazolam over diazepam. Only 10% have indicated preference for using diazepam.9

7.1 Benzodiazepines

The two most commonly used benzodiazepines are midazolam (Versed) and diazepam (Valium). **Midazolam** (Versed) is also classified as an anesthetic adjunct and as a short or intermediate acting hypnotic. It depresses subcortical levels in the Central Nervous System, may potentiate γ-aminobutyric acid (GABA), and may act on the limbic system and reticular formation. It is used for preoperative sedation, anxiety, intubation procedures, induction of general anesthesia, and for diagnostic endoscopic procedures. It can also be used for refractory status epilepticus. For moderate sedation or conscious sedation during endoscopic procedures such as colonoscopy, midazolam can be used alone or in combination with a narcotic (e.g. an analgesic like meperidine or fentanyl). It is administered immediately prior to the procedure and supplemented by small incremental doses throughout until the desired effect is achieved to complete the procedure.[21]

Usual dosing for a healthy adult below 60 years of age range from 1mg to 2.5mg titrated slowly (within 2 minutes). Allow a 2-3 minute interval or more before administering any additional doses, and after each incremental dose to fully evaluate the desired sedative effect. A total dose greater than 5mg is usually not necessary and patients given an additional narcotic may only require 30% less of this drug, because of the cumulative CNS depressant effect (Product Info midazolam hcl injection, 2005). Patients 60 years and older, chronically ill, debilitated or with renal or hepatic insufficiency will require less, 1mg to 1.5mg titrated slowly intravenously (maximum infusion rate is 0.75mg/min). Again, allow 2 or more minutes before each additional dose to evaluate the desired sedative effect. A total dose of greater than 3.5mg is not necessary and individuals will normally require 50% less than what a normal healthy adult would receive especially if a narcotic were also added. An elderly patient should not receive a dose of more than 1.5mg. The peak effect of the drug may take longer and the danger of apnea or hypoventilation is greater. Metabolites of midazolam can accumulate in patients with renal and hepatic failure and may prolong the sedative effect. Administration of midazolam is contraindicated in patients with hypersensitivity to any component of the drug, hypersensitivity to midazolam, acute narrow-angle glaucoma, untreated open-angle glaucoma, pregnancy, and status asthmaticus.[32]

Midazolam is 97% protein bound; has a half-life of 1.8-6.4 hours; metabolized in the liver; excreted in the urine; and crosses the placenta and blood-brain barriers. Given intravenously, it has an onset of 1-5min, for a duration of 1-3 hours. Side effects of the drug include: headache, anxiety, insomnia, retrograde amnesia, euphoria, confusion, agitation, paresthesia, slurred speech, agitation, chills, arrhythmias, nausea, vomiting, hiccups, increased salivation, urticaria, swelling and/or itchiness at injection site, and coughing. Serious adverse effects of the drug include: apnea, cardio-respiratory arrest (occurs usually in combination with a narcotic), oxygen desaturation, hypotension, respiratory depression, respiratory obstruction, bronchospasm and laryngospasm. Unopened vials are stored at room temperature (between 68-77 degrees Fahrenheit or 20-25 degrees Celsius) and are stable up to 36 days. Protect from light.[32] Over sedation can be reversed with the administration of 0.2 mg IV flumazenil (Romazicon, Anexate).

Diazepam (Valium) works similarly as midazolam. It is a member of the following classes: antianxiety, anticonvulsant, benzodiazepine, and long-acting skeletal muscle relaxant. It potentiates the actions of γ-aminobutyric acid (GABA), especially in the limbic system and reticular formation; enhances presympathetic inhibition, and inhibits spinal polysynaptic afferent paths. It is used for anxiety, acute alcohol withdrawal, as an adjunct in seizure disorders; as a relaxant both preoperatively and general skeletal muscle relaxation (adjunct for skeletal muscle spasm). Given rectally, it is used in acute repetitive (refractory) seizures. Other uses of diazepam are: for agitation, benzodiazepine withdrawal, chloroquine overdose, insomnia, and as seizure prophylaxis.[32] For sedation during endoscopic procedures, a dose of 10 mg or less is given intravenously prior to the procedure for a maximum dose of 20 mg. Patients 60 years and older, chronically ill, debilitated or with hepatic insufficiency will require less. There are no specific dose adjustments in patients with renal insufficiency. Due to the irritating nature of the drug, administration **must be done slowly**, no faster than 5mg/min., and if given through IV infusion tubing, give as close to the IV insertion site as possible. Do not inject into small veins (irritating and may cause phlebitis) or through intravenous sets made of polyvinyl chloride (PVC). Diazepam binds to polyvinyl chloride.[32]

Contraindications to its administration are severe hepatic insufficiency, hypersensitivity to diazepam, myasthenia gravis, acute narrow-angle glaucoma, severe respiratory insufficiency, sleep apnea, and children less than 6 months of age. Diazepam is 99% protein bound (and significantly greater in males than in females), metabolized extensively in the liver and excreted in the urine. It is excreted in breast milk, crosses the placenta and blood-brain barriers. It has a half-life of 30-60 hours. Given intravenously, it has an immediate effect and has a duration of about 15 minutes to an hour. Side effects are similar to midazolam and include: dizziness, drowsiness, confusion, headache, anxiety, tremors, stimulation, fatigue, depression, insomnia, hallucinations, ataxia, hypotension, ECG changes and tachycardia. Some, especially for prolonged users, experience blurred vision, tinnitus, mydriasis, nystagmus, constipation, dry mouth, nausea, vomiting, diarrhea, anorexia, neutropenia, rash, dermatitis, and itching. Injectable diazepam can be stored at room temperature and has been found to maintain stability up to 5 months; otherwise, store at temperatures 25 degree Celsius (77°F) or lower to prevent deterioration.

Both diazepam and midazolam are similar in producing effective sedation prior to short surgical as well as endoscopic procedures. However, midazolam produced a greater degree of amnesia, lesser pain on injection, and lesser phlebitis at injection site than diazepam. It also produced a greater respiratory depression than diazepam during the first 45minutes of administration, though the latter sustained the effects longer than midazolam after an hour of administration. Midazolam was also more acceptable to patients than those given diazepam. Hence, midazolam is now the agent of choice when amnesia and adequate sedation is required. One disadvantage, though, noted with the administration of benzodiazepines is that since they are fat-soluble (particularly diazepam), repeated dose results in accumulation of the drug in the adipose tissues which is subsequently released into the bloodstream resulting in prolonged effects. Hence, the most common reasons for missing work were feeling weak and drowsy or having abdominal cramping and bloating.[22] Over sedation can be reversed with the administration of 0.2mg IV flumazenil (Romazicon, Anexate).

7.2 Opiates

The sedative and amnesic effects of benzodiazepines often times do not provide adequate comfort for patients undergoing endoscopic procedures, especially if the procedure lasts longer than half-an-hour. For this reason, opiates are often added to achieve optimum sedation and analgesia. Very few studies have been done to evaluate the efficacy of adding an opiate prior to colonoscopy and authors have casted doubt on its benefit.[8,10,17] The two commonly used opiates are meperidine (Demerol) and fentanyl.

Meperidine (Demerol) is an analgesic, anesthetic adjunct, and is an opioid. It is indicated as an anesthetic adjunct, for obstetrical pain, and as premedication for a procedure. It depresses pain impulses at the spinal cord level by interacting with opioid receptors. For endoscopic procedures, meperidine is dosed as follows: initial bolus of 25mg (given slowly) and subsequent incremental doses of 25mg every 2-3 minutes until the desired effect is achieved. Colonoscopy is usually started two to three minutes after the initial bolus of meperidine and midazolam and titration delivery was given every three minutes thereafter with meperidine 25mg and midazolam 1mg until the desired sedation effect was achieved, i.e. ptosis, slurred speech, and sleep. See Table 2 for dosing guidelines.

Meperidine is readily absorbed and crosses the blood-brain and placental barriers. It is 65-80% protein bound, metabolized in the liver and excreted in the kidneys. It has an elimination half-life of 3.2-3.7 hours. It is contraindicated in individuals with hypersensitivity to meperidine and those who are taking MAOI (monoamine oxidase inhibitor) drugs. Use with caution in individuals with low blood volume, receiving concomitant CNS depressants (reduce dosage), head injury, impaired respiratory function, acute abdominal conditions, Addison's disease (reduce dosage), elderly, debilitated, hypothyroidism, prostatic hypertrophy and urethral strictures, seizures (may induce more), severe hepatic and renal impairment, cardiac dysrhythmias such as SVTs and A-flutter. Side effects include: CNS: drowsiness, dizziness, confusion, headache, sedation, euphoria, increased intracranial pressure, seizures and serotonin syndrome; CV: palpitations, bradycardia, hypotension and orthostatic hypotension, tachycardia; EENT: tinnitus, blurred vision, miosis, diplopia, depressed corneal reflex; GI: nausea, vomiting, anorexia, constipation, cramps, biliary spasm, and paralytic ileus; GU: urinary retention, dysuria; Integ: rash, urticarial, bruising, flushing, diaphoresis, xerostomia and pruritus. Adverse effects include respiratory depression, cardiac arrest and anaphylaxis. Use judiciously when used in conjunction with benzodiazepines because of its added CNS and respiratory depressant effects.[32]

The other opioid of choice is **fentanyl** which shares the same classification as meperidine: analgesic, anesthetic adjunct, and opioid. It acts by inhibiting the ascending pain pathways in the CNS (central nervous system), increases pain threshold, and alters pain perception by binding to opioid receptors. It is used to control moderate to severe pain, as an adjunct to general and regional anesthesia, and premedication for procedures requiring conscious

sedation, such as colonoscopy. Compared to meperidine, fentanyl has a more rapid onset of action and clearance. It also has a lesser incidence of nausea than meperidine.
For procedural sedation, the suggested doses are 0.5 to 1.5mcg/kg intravenously and repeated every 1 to 3 minutes until the desired sedative effects is achieved. **Administer slowly to prevent rigidity**. It is metabolized by the liver, excreted in the kidneys and breast milk and crosses the placenta. Given intravenously, its onset is immediate, within a minute, peaking in 3-5 minutes for ½-1 hour. It has a half-life of 1 ½-6 hours and is 80% bound to plasma proteins. Side effects are similar to meperidine and include: dizziness, delirium, bradycardia, hypo/hypertension, blurred vision, miosis, nausea, vomiting, constipation, urinary retention, rash, diaphoresis, muscle rigidity, cardio-respiratory depression and/or arrest, and laryngospasm. It is contraindicated in individuals with myasthenia gravis and those with hypersensitivity to opiates, bronchial asthma, paralytic ileus, situations of significant respiratory distress.[32]
Opioids and benzodiazepines combined work synergistically. Antagonists of these medications are naloxone (Narcan) for opiates (typical dose is 40-400mcg IV) and flumazenil (Romazicon) for benzodiazepines (typical dose is 40-400mcg IV). These drugs should be readily available in every GI suite to rescue a patient who has been given too much sedative and whose cardiorespiratory status is compromised.

7.3 General anesthetic

The only drug used in colonoscopy in this category is **propofol** (Diprivan). It produces a dose-dependent CNS depression by activating the GABA receptors. Its principal uses are for the induction and maintenance of anesthesia and sedation in mechanically ventilated patients. It also potentiates the effects on the central nervous system of analgesics and sedatives such as benzodiazepines and barbiturates. It has a rapid onset of sedation, but also marked cardio-respiratory depressant properties. These side effects usually rapidly diminish or reverse with reduction of dose or stopping of administration or infusion of propofol. There has been an increase in its use in endoscopic procedures because of its rapid onset and faster recovery to alertness properties with minimal residual sedative effects, which makes it an attractive alternative to the longer half-life benzodiazepines.[22,11] Do not use within 10 days of intake of monoamine oxidase inhibitors (MAOI). This drug potentiates CNS depression in individuals taking antipsychotic drugs, opioids, skeletal muscle relaxants, St. John's wort and alcohol.[32]
Propofol may be used alone or in combination with other agents such an opioid or benzodiazepine. When used alone, higher doses are often required to achieve the desired sedation level which increases the risks of dose-related side effects such as hypotension, respiratory depression, and bradycardia. In combination with other agents, the clinician can adjust the dosages which usually results in administration of smaller dosages of each of the agents to achieve moderate sedation level. If necessary, the effects of the opioid and benzodiazepine can be reversed with naloxone and flumazenil. Propofol does not have an antidote or reversal agent as its half-life is short and the effects wear off as soon as the infusion of the drug is stopped.[9]
Though theoretically, propofol in combination with an opioid or benzodiazepine will decrease the rapid recovery benefit seen with administration of propofol alone, a randomized control trial proved otherwise. The results showed a shorter recovery time with the combination regimen than the propofol alone.[35]

The drug is highly lipophilic. There are two preparations that exist on the market. One is prepared as an oil/water emulsion (Diprivan) consisting of 1% propofol, 10% soybean oil, 2.25% glycerol, 1.2% egg lecithin and the antimicrobial agent, EDTA. This preparation is contraindicated in individuals with propofol, soy or egg hypersensitivities or allergies. The other generic preparation has bisulfites (sodium metabisulfite) as the antimicrobial agent and is therefore, contraindicated in individuals with hypersensitivity or allergy to bisulfites.[4,32]

Propofol is notorious for being painful at the injection site, often described as a burning sensation. Several approaches have been employed to minimize this discomfort. One is the administration of 1-2 ml of 1% lidocaine prior to injecting propofol or mixing lidocaine and propofol in the same syringe. Another approach is diluting propofol in a 5% glucose solution. A study found that there was less pain at the injection site in individuals given the generic propofol (bisulfite-containing propofol) than those given Diprivan.[32]

Propofol is a category B drug and should be used with caution in lactating mothers as it is excreted in breast milk. It is 98% plasma-protein bound, is metabolized primarily in the liver, and excreted in the kidneys. Usual time from injection to onset of sedation is anywhere from 13-30 seconds and the duration is about 4-8 minutes.[4] Table 4 shows a summary of commonly used drugs in colonoscopy.

Drug (Trade Name)	Class	Effects	Dosing Guidelines	Onset/ Peak	Duration/ Half-life	Adverse Effects
Meperidine (Demerol)	Opioid Anesthetic adjunct Analgesic	Sedation Anal-gesia	Bolus 25mg slowly and incremental doses of 25 mg every 2-3 min. titrated to effect	5 min./ Peaks in 10 min.	2-4 hrs. / Half-life of 3-5 hrs.	Respiratory depression, seizures, hypotension, nausea, vomiting tachycardia, and hypoventilation, SVTs confusion, euphoria
Midazolam (Versed)	Benzodia-zepine Anesthetic adjunct Short or intermediate hypnotic	Sedation Amnesia Anxi-olytic	Bolus 0.5-2mg with incremental doses of 2-5mg every 2-3 min titrated to effect	1-5 min./ Peaks in 3-5 min.	1-3 hrs. / Half-life of 1.8-6.4 hrs.	Apnea, hypotension, hypoventilation, cardiac arrhythmias (PVCs), bronchospasm, anxiety, laryngospasm, dyspnea, respiratory depression, headache, agitation

Drug (Trade Name)	Class	Effects	Dosing Guidelines	Onset/ Peak	Duration/ Half-life	Adverse Effects
Diazepam (Valium)	Benzo-diazepine Antianxiety Anticon-vulsant Long-acting skeletal muscle relaxant	Amnesia Anxi-olytic Sedation	Bolus **slowly** 2.5-10mg IV, maximum of 20mg (Do not mix or dilute w/other drugs or solutions in syringe)*	1-5 min./ Peaks in 8 min.	15 min. to 1 hr./ Half-life 30-60 hrs and increases with age and obesity (79-95 hrs.)	Cardiac dysrhythmia, tachycardia, vasculitis, hypotension, respiratory depression, confusion, thrombophlebitis, ataxia, hallucination, tremors, confusion, fatigue, dizziness
Fentanyl (Sublimaze, Fentanyl)	Opioid Anesthetic adjunct Analgesic	Analgesia Sedation	Bolus with 50-100mcg. Or 0.5-1.5mcg/kg per dose. Additional doses at 0.5-1mcg/kg per dose titrated to effect**	<1 min/ Peaks in 3-5 min. for ½-1hr	30-60min./ 1.5-6 hours	Respiratory depression, hypoventilation, decrease in tidal volume, muscle rigidity, delirium, rash, blurred vision, miosis, bradycardia, diaphoresis, laryngospasm
Propofol (Diprivan, Fresenius, Propoven)	Ultra short-acting hypnotic and sedative	Amnesia Hypnotic Sedation	Initial bolus of 10-60mg; Additional doses titrated to level of sedation required every 20-30 seconds, 0.1-0.2 mg/kg/min	13-30 sec/	4-8 min./ 1-8 min.	Respiratory depression, hypoventilation, apnea seizures, hypotension, bradydysrhythmias, hives, flushing, phlebitis, burning at injection site, cough, hiccups, asystole

*Drug is irritating to the vein, administer slowly
**Administer slowly to prevent rigidity

Table 4. Commonly used sedation drugs in colonoscopy

8. Adjuncts to sedation in colonoscopy

There are several adjuncts to the combination of benzodiazepines and opiates. Among these are: Droperidol, promethazine, and diphenhydramine. These medications potentiate the action of the combined benzodiazepine and opiate and the result may be a deeper level of sedation. Adjuncts are employed when the first-line of sedatives fail to produce the desired level of sedation.

Diphenhydramine, better known as Benadryl, acts on the GI tract, blood vessels, and respiratory system by competing with histamine for H-1 receptor sites, thereby decreasing histamine's actions. It is usually used for allergy symptoms, rhinitis, motion sickness, nonproductive cough, antiparkinsonism, insomnia in children, infant colic, and for nighttime sedation. Effects are heightened in individuals taking MAOIs. Side effects include dizziness, drowsiness, anxiety, fatigue, euphoria, confusion, seizures, blurred vision, hypotension, blurred vision, urinary retention, hemolytic anemia, thrombocytopenia, agranulocytosis, chest tightness, wheezing, and anaphylaxis. Dose is 10-50mg IV. It is metabolized in the liver and excreted by the kidneys. It crosses the placenta and is excreted in breast milk. Its onset is immediate when given IV and the duration is 4-7 hours.[32]

Promethazine (Phenergan) acts the same way as diphenhydramine. Its uses are also similar to diphenhydramine. In addition, it is also used to counteract nausea and for preoperative and postoperative sedation. Side effects are the same as diphenhydramine with the addition of neuroleptic syndrome, neuritis and paresthesia, Dose is 12.5mg-50mg IV. Its onset is 3-5 minutes with duration of 4-12 hours. It is metabolized in the liver and excreted in the kidneys and GI tract.[32]

Dropeidol (Inapsine) is a neuroleptic agent acting on the subcortical level producing sleep and tranquilization. It is used as premedication prior to surgery and induction and maintenance of general anesthesia. It is also used as an antiemetic postoperatively. It is also sometimes used for anxiety and for difficult to sedate individuals undergoing therapeutic endoscopy. However, this drug carries a black box warning from the Food and Drug Administration (FDA) warning users that it can prolong the QT interval and should be avoided in individuals with congestive heart failure (CHF), bradycardia, on diuretics, has cardiac hypertrophy, hypokalemia, hypomagnesemia, and are on drugs that normally prolong the QT interval. It is contraindicated in males whose QT intervals are >440msec. or for females whose QT intervals are > 450msec. Individuals over the age of 65, history of alcohol abuse, and use of benzodiazepines and opiates are also at risk. Side effects include seizures, neuroleptic malignant syndrome, torsade de pointes, prolonged QT interval, tachycardia, hypotension, hallucination, depression, extra pyramidal symptoms (EPS), laryngospasm, bronchospasm, chills, and sweating. Initial dose should start at 1.25mg IV. May give an additional 1.25mg IV dose to max of 2.5mg. Its onset is 3-5 min, peaking in ½ an hour and duration of 3-6 hours. It is metabolized in the liver, excreted in the urine and crosses the placenta. It has a half-life of 2-3 hours.[32]

The long duration of actions of these adjuncts make it a less ideal drug for use in short procedures such as colonoscopy. Recovery will take a longer time and will not be cost effective for the GI unit.

9. Conclusion

Colonoscopy remains the gold standard in diagnosing gastrointestinal disorders. The test itself along with the preparation is anxiety provoking and frightening for most people. In many countries around the world, colonoscopy is commonly performed without sedation. The discomfort hampers completion of the test; hence, sedation is now the standard practice in endoscopic procedures, particularly colonoscopy. Benzodiazepines, opiates, and propofol are the commonly used sedating agents. Alone or in combination, many of these agents have been employed to maximize patient comfort and patient and physician satisfaction, but none have proved ideal. The widespread variation in sedation practices are also influenced by physician experience and expertise, financial and regulatory constraints, patient expectations and satisfaction, and lack of consensus on the ideal sedating agent for colonoscopy. More controlled clinical trials are needed to evaluate the safety and efficacy of the ideal sedating agent (s).

10. Acknowledgement

The author wishes to thank Kira Hulse, BS for her review and critique of the article and to Marian de la Cour, RN, BSN, MLS for all her efforts in obtaining most of the articles cited in this chapter and also for her review of this article.

11. References

[1] Aisenberg, J., Brill, J., Ladabaum, U. & Cohen, L. (2005, May). Sedation for gastrointestinal endoscopy: New practices, new economics. *American Journal of Gastroenterology*, 100(5), 996-1000, ISSN 0002-9270.

[2] American Society of Anesthesiologists (2009, October). Standards and guidelines: Distinguishing monitored anesthesia care from moderate sedation/analgesia (Conscious sedation). Retrieved on March 10, 2011 from http://www.asahq.org/For-Healthcare-Professionals/Standards-Guidelines-and-Statements.aspx

[3] American Society of Anesthesiology Task Force on Sedation and Analgesia by Non-anesthesiologists (2002, April). *Anesthesiology*, 96(4), 1004-1017. ISSN 0003-3022.

[4] American Society for Gastrointestinal Endoscopy (ASGE) (2008, November). Sedation and anesthesia in GI endoscopy. *Gastrointestinal Endoscopy*, 68(5), 815-826, ISSN 0016-5107.

[5] Arrowsmith, J., Gertsman, B., Fleischer, D. et al. (1991, July/August). Results from the American Society for Gastrointestinal endoscopy/US Food and Drug Administration collaborative study on complication rates and drug use during gastrointestinal endoscopy. *Gastrointestinal Endoscopy*, 37(4), 421-427, ISSN 0016-5107.

[6] Balsells, F., Wyllie, R., Kay, M. & Steffen, R. (1997, May). Use of conscious sedation for lower and upper gastrointestinal endoscopic examinations in children, adolescents, and young adults: A twelve year review. *Gastrointestinal*

[7] Chung, F. (1995, November). Discharge criteria-a new trend. *Canadian Journal of Anesthesia*, 45(11), 1056-1058. *Endoscopy*, 45(5), 375-380, ISSN 0016-5107.

[8] Cohen, l., Delegge,M., Aisenberg, J. et al. (2007). AGA Institute review of endoscopic sedation. *Gastroenterology*, 133, 675-701, ISSN 0016-5085.

[9] Cohen, L.,Wecsler, L., Gaetano, J. et. al. (2006, May). Endoscopic sedation in the United States: Results from a nationwide survey. *American Journal of Gastroenterology*, 101(5), 967-974, ISSN 0002-9270.

[10] Cohen, L., Hightower, C., Wood, D. et al. (2004, June). Moderate level sedation during colonoscopy: A prospective study using low-dose propofol, meperidine/fentanyl, and midazolam. *Gastrointestinal Endoscopy*, 59(7), 795-803, ISSN 0016-5107.

[11] Deenadayalu, V., Eid, E., Goff, J. et al. (2008). Non-anesthesiologist administered propofol sedation for endoscopic procedures: A worldwide safety review (abstract). *Gastrointestinal Endoscopy*, 67, AB107.

[12] Froehlich, F., Harris, J., Wietlisbach, V., et al. (2006, May). Current sedation and monitoring practice for colonoscopy: An international observational study (EPAGE). *Endoscopy*, 38(5), 461-469. ISSN 0013-726x.

[13] Godwin, S., Caro, D., Wolf, S. et al. (2005, February). Clinical policy: Procedural sedation and analgesia in the emergency department. *Annals of Emergency Medicine*, 45(2), 177-196. ISSN 0196-0644.

[14] Gross, B., Bailey, P., Connis, R. et al (2002, April.) Practice guidelines for sedation and analgesia by non-anesthesiologists. *Anesthesiology*, 96(4), 1004-1017, ISSN 0003-3022.

[15] Heuss, L., Froehlich, F. & Beglinger, C. (2005, May). Changing patterns of sedation and monitoring practice during endoscopy: Results of a nationwide survey in Switzerland. *Endoscopy*, 37(5), 161-166. ISSN 013-726x.

[16] Huang, R. & Eisen, G. (2004, April). Efficacy, safety, and limitations in current practice of sedation and analgesia. *Gastrointestinal Endoscopy Clinics of North America*, 14(2), 269-288. ISSN 1052-5157.

[17] Jung, H., Bae, K., Yoon, S. et al. (2004, February). Comparison of midazolam versus midazolam/meperidine during colonoscopy in a prospective, randomized, double-blind study. *Korean Journal of Gastroenterology*, 43(2), 96-103, ISSN 1598-9992.

[18] Kissin, I., (2000, May). Depth of anesthesia and Bispectral Index Monitoring. *Anesthesia & Analgesia*, 90(5), 1114-1117, ISSN 003-2999.

[19] Kubilay, Ç., Yakut, M. & Özden, A. (2009, December). Sedation with midazolam versus midazolam plus meperidine for routine colonoscopy: A prospective, randomized , controlled study. *Turkish Journal of Gastroenterology*, 20(4), 271-275, ISSN 1300-4948.

[20] Külling, D., Orlandi, M. & Inauen, W. (2007, September). Propofol sedation during endoscopic procedures: How much staff and monitoring are necessary? *Gastrointestinal Endoscopy*, 66(3), 443-449, ISSN 0016-5107.

[21] Lee, H. & Kim, J. H. (2009, August 14). Superiority of split dose midazolam as conscious sedation for outpatient colonoscopy. *World Journal of Gastroenterology*, 15(30), 3783-3787, ISSN 1007-9327.

[22] Lubarsky, D., Candiotti, K & Harris, E. (2007, August). Understanding modes of moderate sedation during gastrointestinal procedures: A current review of the literature. *Journal of Clinical Anesthesia*, 19(5), 397-404. ISSN 0952-8180.

[23] McQuaid, K. & Laine, L. (2008, May). A systematic review and meta-analysis of randomized, controlled trials of moderate sedation for routine endoscopic procedures. *Gastrointestinal Endoscopy*, 67(6), 910-922, ISSN 0016-5107. Mosby's Nursing Drug Reference

[24] Ong, W., Santosh, D., Lakhtakia, S. & Reddy. (2007, September). A randomized, controlled trial on use of propofol alone versus propofolwith midazolam, ketamine, and pentazocine "sedato-analgesic cocktail" for sedation during ERCP. *Endoscopy*, 39(9),807-812. ISSN 0013-726x.

[25] Padmanabhan, U., Leslie, K., SingYi Eer, A. et al. (2009, November). Early cognitive impairment after sedation for colonoscopy: The effect of adding midazolam and/or fentanyl to propofol. *Anesthesia & Analgesia*, 109(5), 1448-1455 ISSN 0003-2999.

[26] Padmanabhan, U. & Leslie, K. (2008, May)). Australian anesthetists' practice of sedation for gastrointestinal endoscopy in adult patients. *Anaesthesia and Intensive Care*, 36(3), 436-441.

[27] Qadeer, M.,Vargo, J., Khandala, F. et al (2005, November). Propofol versus traditional sedative agents for gastrointestinal endoscopy: Ameta-analysis. *Clinical Gastroenterology and Hepatology*, 3(11), 1049-1056. ISSN1542-3565.
[28] Rex, D. & Khalfan, H. (2005, October). Sedation and the technical performance of colonoscopy. *Gastrointestinal Endoscopy Clinics of North America*, 15(4), 661-672. ISSN 1052-5157.
[29] Rex, D., Overley, C., Kinser, K. et al. (2002, May). Safety of propofol administration by registered nurses with gastroenterologist supervision in 2000 endoscopic cases. *American Journal of Gastroenterology*, 97(5), 1159-1163, ISSN 0002-9270.
[30] Seifert, H., Schmitt, T., Gültekin, T., Caspary, W. & Wehrmann, T. (2000, September). Sedation with propofol plus midazolam versus propofol alone for interventional endoscopic procedures: A prospective, randomized study. *Alimentary Pharmacology & Therapeutics*, 14(9), 1207-1214, ISSN 1365-2036.
[31] The Merriam-Webster Dictionary (1997). Springfield, MA USA, ISBN 0-87779-911-3.
[32] Tohda, G., Higashi, S., Wakahara, S. et al. (2006,April). Propofol sedation during endoscopic procedures: Safe and effective administration by registered nurses supervised by endoscopists. *Endoscopy*, 38(4), 360-367. ISSN 0013-726x.
[33] Tohda, G., Higashi, S., Sakumoto, H., et al. (2006, July). Efficacy and safety of nurse-administered propofol sedation during emergency upper endoscopy for gastrointestinal bleeding: A prospective study. *Endoscopy*, 38(7), 684-689, ISSN 0013-726x.
[34] VanNatta, M. & Rex, D. (2006). Propofol alone titrated to deep sedation versus propofol in combination with opioids and/or benzodiazepines and titrated to moderate sedation for colonoscopy. *American Journal of Gastroenterology*, 101, 2209-2217, ISSN 0002-9270.
[35] Vargo, J., Bramley, T., Meyer, K. et al. (2007, July). Practice efficiency and economics: The case for rapid recovery sedation agents for colonoscopy in a screening population. *Journal of Clinical Gastroenterology*, 41(6), 591-598. ISSN 0192-0790.
[36] Vargo, J., Zuccaro, G.,Dumot, J., et al. (2002, July). Gastroenterologist-administered propofol versus meperidine and midazolam for advanced upper endoscopy: A prospective, randomized trial. *Gastroenterology*, 123(1), 8-16, ISSN 0016-5085.
[37] Waring, J., Baron, T., Hirota, W. et al. (2003, September). Guidelines for conscious sedation and monitoring during gastrointestinal endoscopy. *Gastrointestinal Endoscopy*, 58(3), 317-322, ISSN 0016-5107.
[38] Wehrmann, T. & Riphaus, A. (2009, January). Sedation, surveillance, and preparation. *Endoscopy*, 41(1), 86-90. ISSN 0013-726x.
[39] White, P., Fanzca, S. & Dajun, S. (1999). New criteria for fast-tracking after out-patient anesthesia: A comparison with the Modified Aldrete's Scoring System, *Anesthesia & Analgesia*, 88, 1069-1072, ISSN 0003-2999.
[40] Shao, X., Hong, L., White, P., et al (2000, May). Bisulfite-containing propofol: Is it a cost-effective alternative to Diprivan for induction of anesthesia? *Anesthesia & Analgesia*, 91, 871-875, ISSN 0003-2999.
[41] Zavoral, M., Suchanek, S., Zavada, F. et al. (2009, December 21). Colorectal cancer screening in Europe. *World Journal of Gastroenterology*, 15(47), 5907-5915, ISSN 1007-9327.

5

The Diagnostic Value of Colonoscopy in Understanding Inflammatory Mucosal Damage in Patients with Ulcerative Colitis and Predicting Clinical Response to Adsorptive Leucocytapheresis as a Non-Pharmacologic Treatment Intervention

Tomotaka Tanaka[1], Abbi R Saniabadi[2] and Yasuo Suzuki[3]
[1]*Akitsu Prefectural Hospital, Akitsu cho, Hiroshima,*
[2]*Department of Pharmacology, Hamamatsu University School of Medicine, Hamamatsu*
[3]*Department of Internal Medicine, Sakura Medical Centre, Toho University, Chiba*
Japan

1. Introduction

The gastrointestinal system consists of a hollow muscular tube starting from the oral cavity, where food enters the mouth, continuing through the pharynx, oesophagus, stomach and intestines to the rectum and anus, where faeces pass out. The primary purpose of the gastrointestinal system is to break down food into nutrients, which together with water can be absorbed to feed the body cells. In the case of gastrointestinal disease or disorders, these functions of the gastrointestinal tract are not achieved successfully, discussed in the subsequent sections of this chapter. The innermost layer of the gastrointestinal system is the mucosa, which is lined with specialised epithelial cells, supported by an underlying connective tissue layer called the lamina propria, where infiltrating leucocytes, in particular, myeloid linage leucocytes are often seen.

2. The natural history of ulcerative colitis

Ulcerative colitis (UC) is one of the two major phenotypes of the idiopathic inflammatory bowel diseases (IBD) of the intestine; the other major phenotype is Crohn's disease (CD). UC and CD are both debilitating chronic disorders that afflict millions of individuals throughout the world with symptoms which impair function and quality of life. However, whereas UC is confined to the colon and the rectum, CD may affect any part of the gut from the mouth to the perianal (1,2). A multitude of clinical manifestations represent the expressions of IBD. These include diarrhoea, rectal bleeding, abdominal discomfort, fever, anaemia, and weight loss; both UC and CD tend to run a remitting-relapsing course affected by diverse environmental factors (2). From here on, we shall focus only on UC. The severity of UC is often presented by clinical activity index (CAI). Another, but complementary parameter is endoscopic activity index, not used in this chapter.

3. Colonoscope, the gastroenterologist's eye and arms in modern times

Colonoscopy is a revolutionary development in gastroenterology, now days like both arm and eyes for specialist gastroenterologists that can reach the inside of the large and distal segment of the small intestine. Introduced in the late 1960s (3), the term, colonoscopy refers to the endoscopic examination of the bowel with a charge-coupled device (CCD) camera or a fiber optic camera on a flexible tube passed through the rectal opening. As the name implies, colonoscopy allows a visual diagnosis of intestinal wall lesions like inflammation, ulceration, polyps and provides the opportunity for biopsy or removal of suspected cancerous lesions. Colonoscopy can remove polyps as small as one millimetre or less. Once polyps are removed, they can be studied with the aid of a microscope to determine if they are precancerous or not. Retrograde colonoscopy of the entire colon, and endoscopic excision of polyps from anywhere in the colon, began in 1969 (4). Momentous advances have occurred over the past two decades, and the two procedures are now widely accepted and practiced. Development and perfection of the methodology were, at first, fraught with many difficulties, both procedural and technical, which had to be overcome. Significant opposition was engendered in the early years by some who claimed that the methods were both unnecessary and unduly dangerous. Time has proven otherwise. Progress came about as the result of a steady stream of publications from a number of centres documenting the successful and safe application of the methodology.

More advanced versions include virtual colonoscopy, which uses 2D and 3D imagery reconstructed from computed tomography (CT) scans or from nuclear magnetic resonance (MR) scans, is also possible, as a totally non-invasive medical test. However, unlike standard colonoscopy, virtual colonoscopy does not allow for therapeutic maneuvers such as polyp/tumour removal or biopsy nor visualization of lesions smaller than 5 millimeters. If a growth or polyp is detected by using CT colonography, a standard colonoscopy would still need to be performed. Further, colonoscopy is similar to, but not the same as, sigmoidoscopy, the difference being related to which parts of the colon each can examine. A colonoscopy allows an examination of the entire colon (measuring more than 1.5m in length). A sigmoidoscopy allows an examination of only the final 60cm of the colon. A sigmoidoscopy is often used as a screening procedure for a full colonoscopy to be followed in many instances in conjunction with a faecal occult blood test, which can detect the formation of cancerous cells throughout the colon. At other times, a sigmoidoscopy is preferred to a full colonoscopy in patients having an active flare of ulcerative colitis (UC) or Crohn's disease (CD) to avoid a perforation of the colon. Additionally, surgeons use the term pouchoscopy to refer to a colonoscopy of the ileo-anal pouch. Conditions that call for diagnostic colonoscopy include gastrointestinal haemorrhage, unexplained changes in bowel habit and suspicion of malignancy. Colonoscopies are often used to diagnose colon cancer, but are also frequently used to diagnose and assess inflammatory bowel disease (IBD). In older patients (sometimes even younger ones) an unexplained drop in haematocrit (one sign of anaemia) is an indication that calls for a colonoscopy, usually along with an oesophagogastroduodenoscopy, even if no obvious blood has been seen in the stool (faeces).

Due to the high mortality associated with colon cancer and the high effectiveness and low risks associated with colonoscopy, it is now becoming a routine screening test for people 50 years of age or older. Subsequent re-screenings are then scheduled based on the initial results found, with a five or ten-year recall being common for colonoscopies that produce normal results (5). Patients with a family history of colon cancer are often first screened during their teenage years. A recent study found that among people who have had an initial colonoscopy that found no polyps, the risk of developing colorectal cancer within five years is extremely low. Therefore, there is no need for those people to have another colonoscopy sooner than five years after the first screening (6). In this chapter, the authors endeavour to describe the potential diagnostic power of colonoscopy potentially to identify patients with an active flare of UC who are most likely to respond to selective, but therapeutic removal of circulating myeloid linage leucocytes (granulocytes and monocytes/macrophages) by extracorporeal adsorption, as a new and non-pharmacologic treatment intervention for patients with IBD, better known as GMA, which stands for granulocyte and monocyte adsorption (7).

4. Colonoscopy in inflammatory bowel diseases

Figure 1 shows colonoscopy photographs from the surface of the colonic mucosa of healthy human subjects or patients with UC following full remission in association with GMA therapy. The mucosa is the surface through, which nutrients and water from the food in the intestine are absorbed into the blood stream. Accordingly, healthy mucosa is typically well vascularised for adequate absorption. Colonoscopy has a unique position in viewing and assessing intestinal integrity.

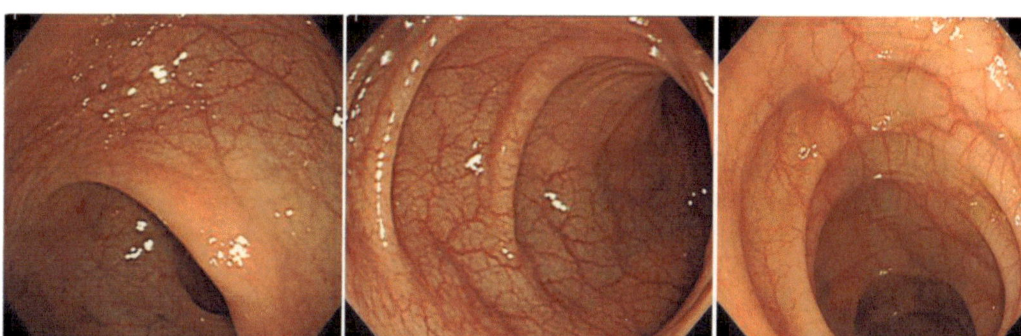

Fig. 1.

Most symptoms of UC are due to the ulceration and the loss of the mucosal layer covering the inner wall of the large intestine (colon and the rectum). As the mucosal layer is involved in the absorption of nutrients and water from the gut, during severely active UC, absorption of nutrients and water is seriously impaired. In Figure 2, typical colonoscopy photographs from the surface of the colon or the rectum of patients with severe and fulminant UC are seen. There is extensive and deep ulcers together with near total loss of the mucosal tissue. This condition is debilitating, the patients may suffer from weight loss, and impaired quality of life. For example unabsorbed food and water will pass as watery diarrhoea, or bloody diarrhoea due to bleeding. Such patients are not likely to respond to any drug based medication or even to therapeutic depletion of myeloid leucocytes by GMA, they have fulminant (disease persists in the presence of optimal medication) UC and often must opt for surgery known as colectomy. Needless to say that only an initial diagnostic colonoscopy can identify such patients as non-responders to drug based interventions so that the patient can opt for colectomy at an early stage. This should significantly shorten morbidity time and save medical cost.

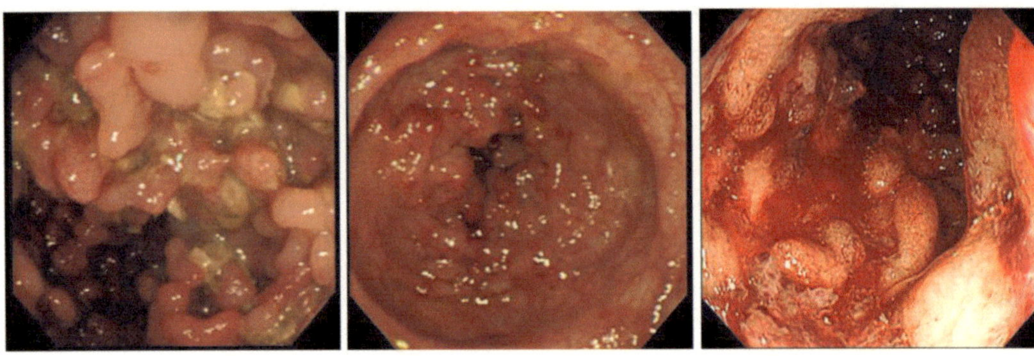

Fig. 2.

5. Therapeutic options for patients with ulcerative colitis

Despite the recognition of a genetic background together with environmental factors, which at present are thought to translate into an inappropriate inflammatory response in patients with UC (2, 8-10), currently our understanding on the immunopathogenesis of UC is inadequate. Hence, up to now drug therapy of UC has been empirical rather than based on sound understanding of disease aetiology. Accordingly, while drug therapy initially appears successful in the majority of patients, it comes at the cost of significant side effects (11,12). Further, up to now, first line medications for exacerbation of UC include 5-aminosalicylic acid (5-ASA) or sulphasalazine in combination with a corticosteroid with consideration of azathioprine (or 6-mercaptopurine) and nutritional support for some patients (2,14-18). Treatment failure in patients with severe disease has often been an indication for colectomy in up to 40% of steroid refractory patients (2,19, 20) although in recent years, cyclosporin A (CsA) has been introduced for corticosteroid refractory UC (18,21). Despite being moderately effective in this clinical setting in reducing colectomy rates, there remain serious concerns over long-term efficacy and toxicity of CsA (22).

However, this is not to say that drug has no place in the treatment of UC. In fact, no one can deny the role of medicines in the elimination of most disease that our ancestors were left defenseless against. However, even in today's era of modern medicine, it is essential to bear in mind that drug therapy by its very nature, involves adding a foreign substance to the body system and although initially effective, may lead to the disease becoming drug dependent or refractory. Additionally, many drugs are associated with toxic side effects which can add to the disease complexity. Hence, a therapeutic strategy based on a non-drug intervention, a correction or support of body's natural processes like GMA (which takes away from the body instead of adding to it), if effective, should have advantages over drugs, long term adverse side effects and refractoriness are unlikely (23, 24).

6. Myeloid leucocytes, cytokines and ulcerative colitis

It is now known that UC is exacerbated by inflammatory cytokines like tumour necrosis factor (TNF)-α, interleukin (IL)-1β, IL-6, IL-8 and others (25). Accordingly, anti-cytokine antibodies, notably anti-TNF antibodies like infliximab (IFX) are being used and new antibodies are being developed for the treatment of IBD (26). Indeed, the efficacy of anti-TNF, notably IFX, in patients with CD (27) as well as in UC (26) has validated the role of this cytokine in the immunopathogenesis of IBD. However, the enthusiasm towards biologicals is increasingly being dampened by concerns about their long-term efficacy and in particular, the safety profiles (28,29). However, patients with active IBD harbour elevated and activated myeloid linage leucocytes (granulocytes and monocytes) in the presence of compromised lymphocytes (1,30-33). Further, histologic examinations of mucosal biopsies from patients with active IBD reveals a spectrum of pathologic manifestations among which an abundance of neutrophils accounts not only for the morphologic lesions in IBD, but also for the prevailing patterns of mucosal inflammation (2,34,35). When activated, myeloid leucocytes produce an array of pleiotropic cytokines like TNF-α, IL-1β, IL-6, IL-12, IL-23, which are strongly pro-inflammatory (25,36). Therefore, targeting leucocytes as key players in the exacerbation of IBD is what lies behind extracorporeal granulocyte monocyte/macrophage adsorption (GMA) with the Adacolumn (7). Likewise, neutrophils in patients with IBD show activation behaviour (30) and prolonged survival time (37). Factors that are known to promote neutrophil survival in IBD include inflammatory cytokines (38) and paradoxically corticosteroids (39), which are commonly used to treat IBD patients. Myeloid leucocytes, like the CD14(+)CD16(+) monocytes are major sources of TNF-α (40,41), and it could be valid to say that selective depletion of myeloid leucocytes by GMA should alleviate inflammation and promote remission or at least enhance the efficacy of pharmacologics. However, clinical studies in patients with UC have reported unmatched efficacy outcomes, ranging from an 85% (42) to a statistically insignificant level (43), indicating that certain subpopulations of patients benefit from GMA while others not so, suggesting that patients' baseline demographic variables determine clinical response to this non-pharmacologic mode of therapy (23,24).

7. Therapeutic leucocytapheresis in ulcerative colitis – logics and mechanisms

For an extracorporeal intervention to be a novel non-drug therapeutic option, it should be able to selectively deplete leucocytes, which in patients with UC are thought to contribute to the disease pathogenesis. For example, we have already said that patients with active IBD are found to have compromised lymphocytes (31-33). With this in mind, certain sub-populations of lymphocytes like the CD4(+)CD25(+) phenotype, known as the regulatory T cells (Treg) have essential immunoregulatory roles and therefore, are indispensable to the host (44-49). Based on these understandings, the Adacolumn leucocytapheresis system is designed to spare lymphocytes. It is filled with specially designed cellulose acetate beads of 2mm in diameter as the column leucocytapheresis carriers that are bathed in physiologic saline (50). The carriers remove from blood in the column most of the granulocytes, monocytes/macrophages together with some platelets (7,51). Surprisingly, the procedure has been associated with a sustained increase in absolute lymphocyte counts in the post treatment phase (32,33,50) including the regulatory phenotype, CD4(+)CD25(+) Treg (7,49,50). The Adacolumn is an adsorptive type and leucocytapheresis with this column is often abbreviated as GMA. The mechanisms for sparing lymphocytes are briefly described here. Patients with immune dysfunction may have immune complexes (IC) in their plasma (7,51,52). Cellulose acetate adsorbs immunoglobulin G (IgG) and IC from the plasma (52,53). Upon adsorption, the binding sites on IgG and IC become available for the Fcγ receptors (FcγRs) on myelocytes (7,51-53). Further, cellulose acetate with adsorbed IgG and IC generates complement activation fragments including C3a and C5a (7,52,53). The opsonins C3b/C3bi and others derived from the activation fragments also adsorb onto the carriers and serve as binding sites for the leucocyte complement receptors, CR1, CR2, CR3 (Mac-1, CD11b/CD18). Hence, leucocyte adsorption to the GMA carriers in the Adacolumn is governed by the opsonins, FcγRs and the leucocytes complement receptors (7,53). The expressions of these sets of receptors are common features of myeloid linage leucocytes. Lymphocytes are not known to express complement receptors except on small subsets of B, T and natural killer (NK) cells. Similarly, FcγRs are not widely expressed on lymphocytes except on small populations of $CD19^{+}$B cells and $CD56^{+}$NK cells (7,51). These basic phenomena proceed well on the carriers and lend the Adacolumn GMA selectivity.

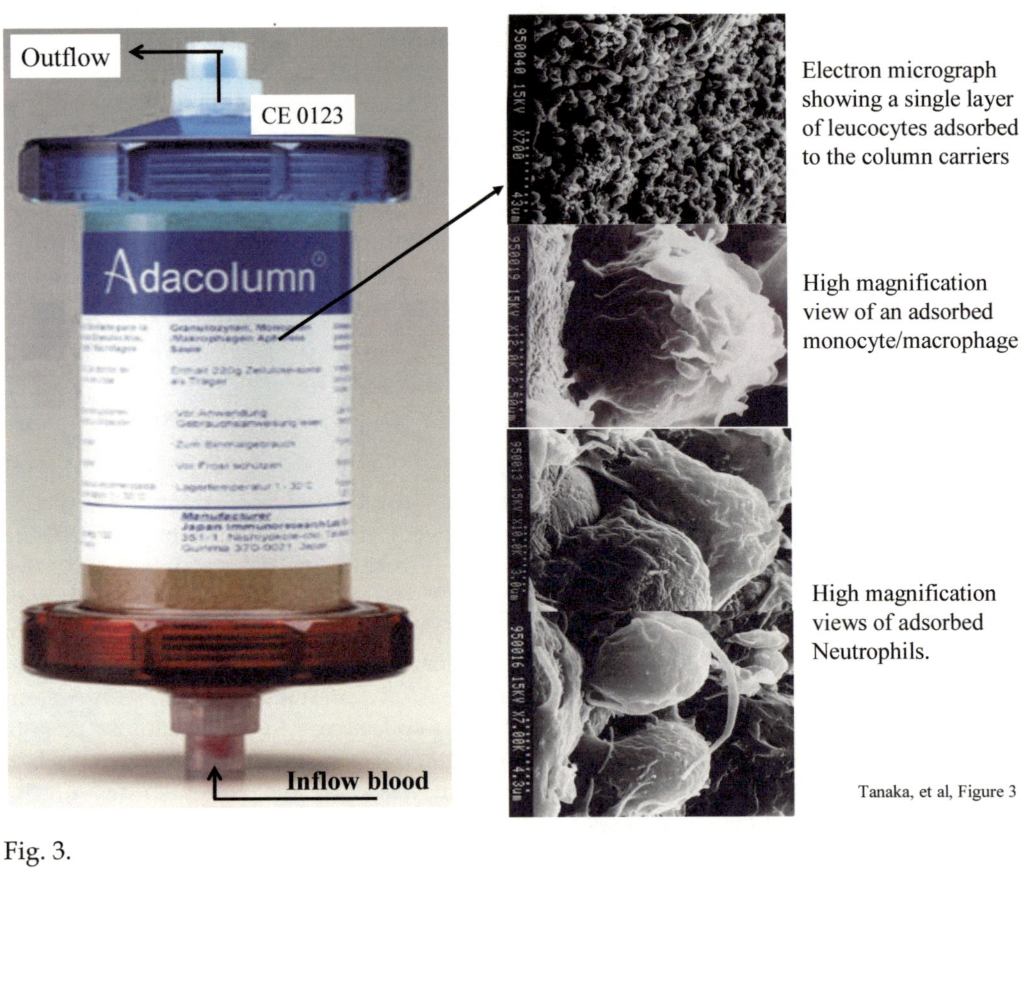

Fig. 3.

8. Colonoscopic features of typical responders to GMA

Clinical experience has shown that GMA in patients with steroid dependent or steroid refractory UC was associated with significant efficacy as assessed by measuring the fall in UC clinical activity index (CAI) and tapering or discontinuation of steroids, while in steroid naïve patients, GMA spared patients from exposure to steroids (23,24). Therefore, published data (23,24,32,34,55) suggest that steroid naive patients respond particularly well. Characteristically they respond faster with fewer GMA sessions and have a high cumulative rate of remission. Thus, the remission rate in steroid naïve patients reported by Suzuki et al. (32) was an 85%. Similarly, Tanaka et al. (34) treated a cohort of 45 patients, 26 steroid naive and 19 steroid dependent. Each patient could receive up to a maximum of 11 GMA sessions (or until CAI decreased to 4 or less). At week 12, the response rate (CAI ≤4) in steroid naïve subgroup was 22 of 26 patients (84.6%) and in steroid dependent sub-group was 11 of 19 (57.9%). Colonoscopy revealed that most non-responders in both groups had deep colonic ulcers and extensive loss of the mucosal tissue. Further, this is the only study that looked at the impact of GMA on leucocyte level in the colonic mucosa. Biopsies taken during colonoscopy revealed massive infiltration of the colonic mucosa by neutrophils and GMA was associated with a striking reduction of neutrophils in the mucosa (Figure 5). Tanaka's colonoscopic observations (23,34) echo those of Suzuki et al. a few years earlier (32), who also reported that the only 3 non-responders in their cohort of 20 steroid naïve patients had deep colonic ulcers. In a very thorough study by Suzuki et al. (56), the authors aimed at determining the responders to GMA. Their major findings are as follows. Seven days after the last GMA session, 20 of 28 patients (71.4%) achieved clinical remission including all 8 patients who had their first UC episode. The mean duration of UC in the 8 first episode

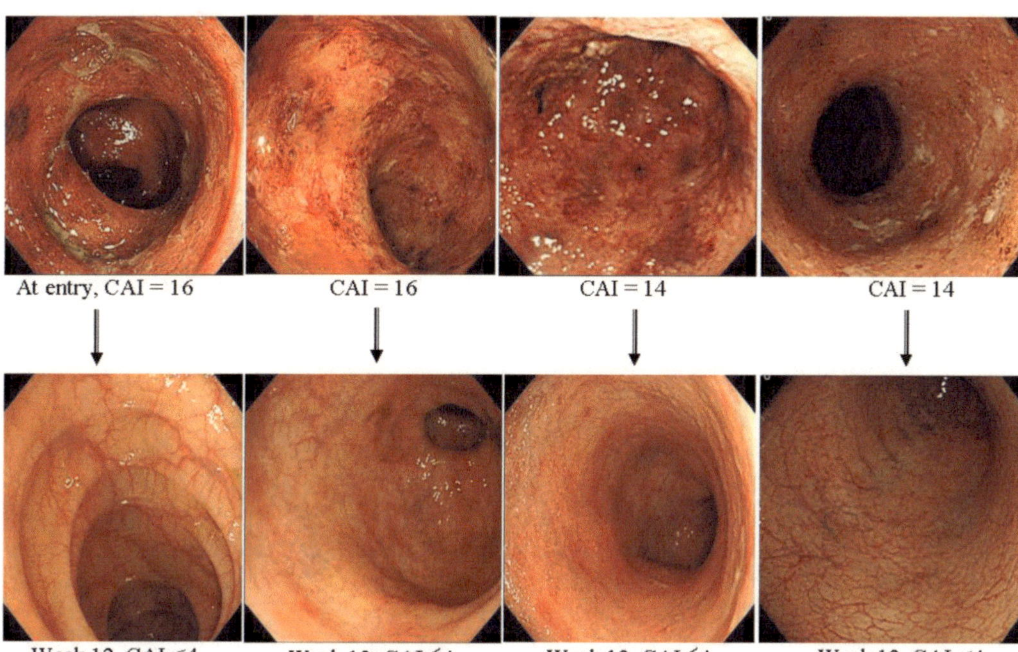

Fig. 4.

cases was just 3.4 months compared with 40.2 months for all 28 patients and 65.4 months for the 8 patients who did not respond at al. The response to GMA seemed to be independent of baseline CAI. The authors concluded that first UC episode and short disease duration might be good predictors of response to GMA in that clinical setting. Further, they stated that GMA could be an effective first line medication for steroid naïve patients (23,32,56).

9. The impact of GMA on mucosal leucocytes

It is of particular interest to see if GMA, in fact does impact the mucosal level of infiltrating myeloid leucocytes. As stated above, colonic biopsies were taken from active disease sites before and after GMA induced remission in patients with active UC. Figure 5 shows representative histology photographs from a GMA responder patient. The specimen taken at baseline shows the colonic mucosa is infiltrated by a vast number of inflammatory leucocytes, primarily granulocytes and monocytes/macrophages; the density of the infiltrating cells was strongest in or around the glandular lumen (crypt abscesses). The specimen taken when the patient had achieved remission shows very striking reduction in inflammatory cell infiltrate. Surprisingly, the density of leucocytes was reported to be stronger in steroid naïve patients vs patients on steroids, suggesting that corticosteroids have inhibitory effects on neutrophils (23).

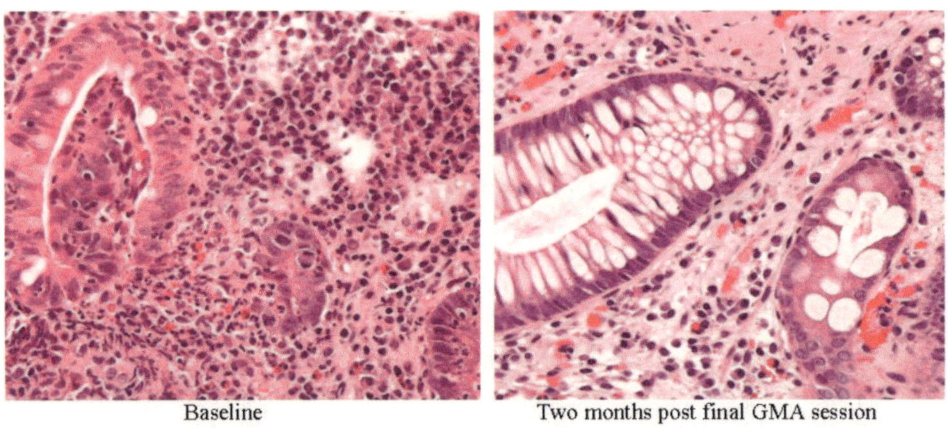

Fig. 5.

10. Colonoscopic features of non-responders to GMA

As reviewed above, several studies have reported that any patient with a fair level of colonic mucosa is a potential responder to GMA. In contrast, Figure 2 (above) shows deep and extensive colonic lesions with virtually no mucosal tissue left at the lesion sites in two typical GMA non-responder patients. Such patients are unlikely to respond to any medication except colectomy. Even patients with a near equal CAI score had very different mucosal damage status, indicating that CAI per se does not reflect the full extent of mucosal damage in patients with UC. Figure 6 shows colonoscopy photographs from the colonic mucosa of a 60-year-old steroid dependent patient who showed partial response to GMA. At baseline, the major colonoscopic findings seen are strong inflammation with multiple polyp-like protrusions in the mucosa. Following a course of GMA therapy, inflammation has alleviated, but multiple polyps are exposed and apparently seem not to be affected by GMA, but the mucosa appears to be regenerating once again, suggesting a fair level of mucosal tissue was left prior to the initiation of GMA therapy. Based on CAI, this patient might be in clinical remission, but has not achieved endoscopic (colonoscopic) remission, which could require a long observation time.

A small minority of patients without deep colonic lesions or extensive loss of the mucosal tissue do not respond to GMA as well. Colonoscopy photographs from such patients are presented in Figure 7, showing inflammation, but without extensive ulcers (entry CAI, 15). These cases are likely to have a long history of multiple drug therapy. However, no patient with the entry colonoscopy features seen in Figure 2 did show any significant fall in CAI score.

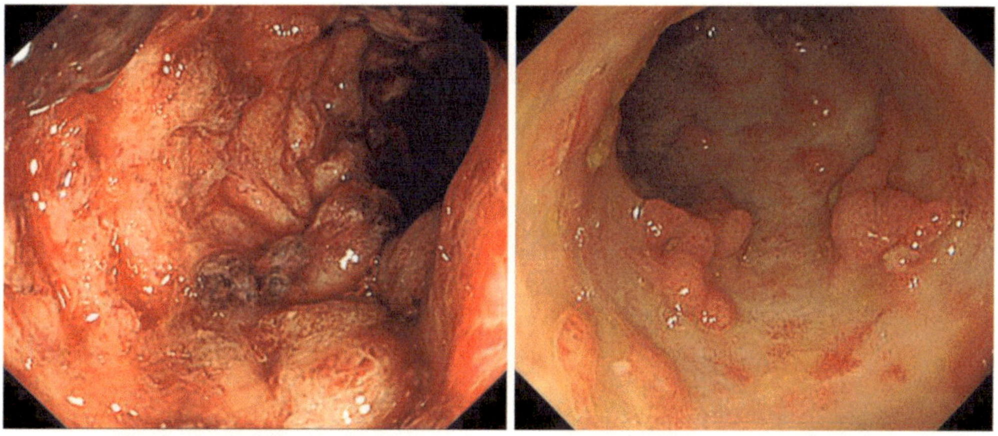

A 60-year-old patient with left-sided colitis, steroid dependent with severe UC in the presence of optimal corticosteroid, baseline CAI = 16.

Four months post last GMA (partial response)

Fig. 6.

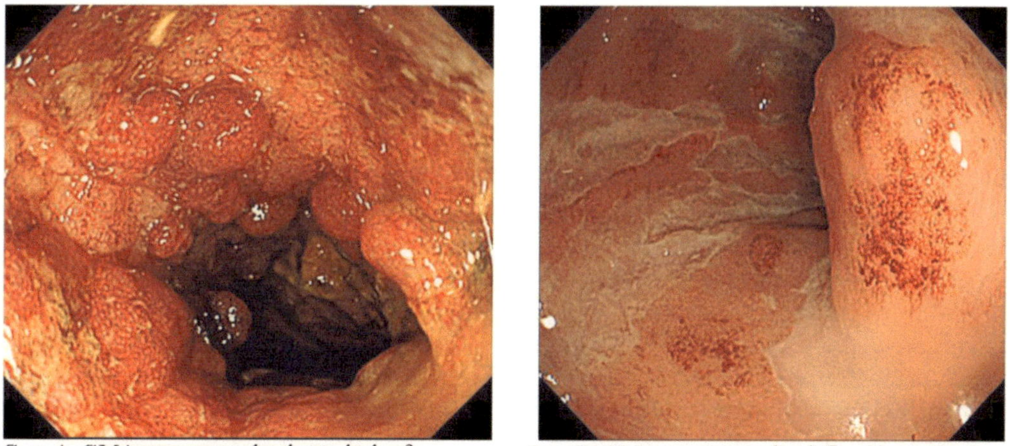

Case A, GMA non-responder due to lack of adequate mucosal tissue.

Case B, GMA non-responder defined by patient's demography

Fig. 7.

11. Colonoscopic features of patients who are most likely to respond to GMA

From the plethora of published clinical observations, it appears that drug naïve patients with superficial lesions, usually first episode cases are the best responders to GMA, respond soon after a few GMA sessions and can be spared from multiple drug therapy. Typical colonoscopic features in these patients are seen in Figure 8. Accordingly, GMA should have maximum impact if applied immediately after a flare up, and be most effective in first episode cases.

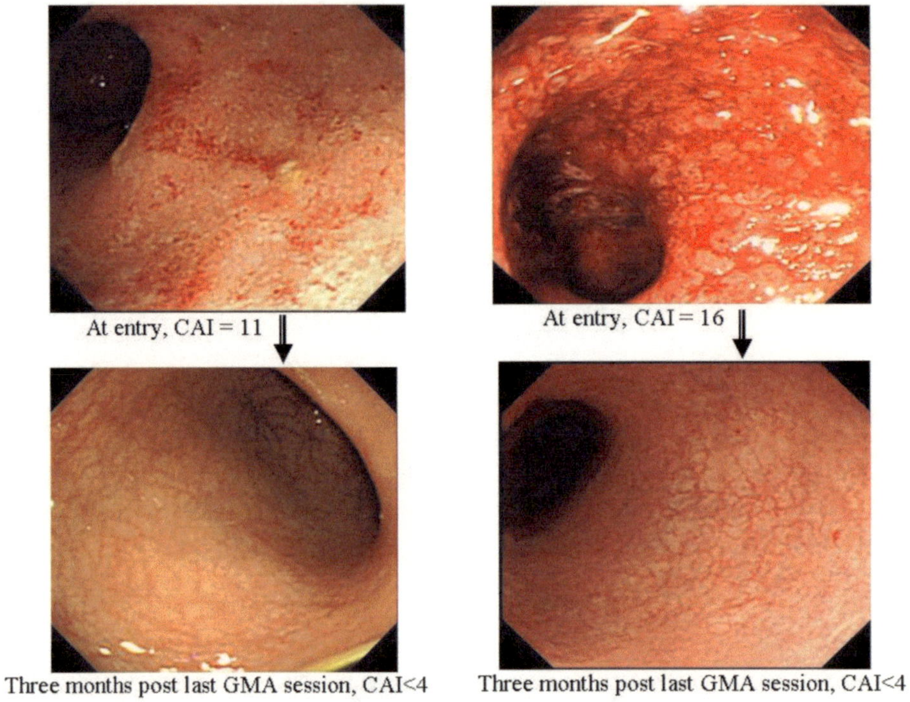

Fig. 8.

12. Concluding remarks

The gastrointestinal system is often affected by diseases which can impair its function and the individual's well being. The colonoscope may be regarded as the gastroenterologist's eyes and arms. Within limits, surgery can be achieved by the application of colonoscope like removing suspected cancerous lesions and excision of polyps which grow inside the large intestine in many individuals and can cause morbidity. Further, the large intestine is the main organ where IBD, in particular UC develops as a very debilitating health disorder. UC patients present with diverse clinical and endoscopic disease severity levels, and therefore, their clinical response to medical interventions can be complete remission, partial response or no response at all. Therefore, without colonoscopic evaluations of patients' relevant demographic variables, medical resources will be wasted together with prolonged morbidity time for many patients. Further, patients with UC have activated myeloid leucocytes, which infiltrate the colonic mucosa in vast numbers and potentially can exacerbate the inflammation and perpetuate the disease. Accordingly, efficient depletion of myeloid leucocytes by GMA, which reduces the mucosal concentrations of myeloid leucocytes, should benefit patients with UC. In spite of this view, clinical efficacy outcomes are both encouraging as well as disappointing; the answer might lie in the patients' disease status at entry. By the power of colonoscopy over a decade in patients with UC we have learnt that all patients with the first UC episode and short duration of disease readily respond to GMA and can be spared from multiple drug therapy. Similarly, most steroid naïve or dependent patients who have a fair level of intact mucosal tissue are potential responders to GMA. Patients with extensive loss of the mucosal tissue and those with a long history of exposure to multiple drugs like corticosteroids are unlikely to respond to GMA. Further, one of the most favoured features of Adacolumn GMA is its safety profile. Serious side effects are very rare. This is in sharp contrast to multiple severe side effects associated with most conventional pharmacologicals and new biologics. Our view is that in patients with UC, there is an evolving scope for therapeutic opportunity based on taking away the sources of inflammatory cytokines.

13. Acknowledgements

The authors received no external funding in connection with the work described in this manuscript. Similarly, the authors have no conflict of interest in relation to the publication of this work.

14. References

[1] Selby W (1997). The natural history of ulcerative colitis. Baillieres Clin Gastroenterol; 11:53-64.
[2] Allison MC, Dhillon AP, Lewis WG, Pounder RE (Eds): Inflammatory Bowel Disease. London: Mosby 1998, pp9-95.
[3] Wolff WI (1989). Colonoscopy: history and development. Am J Gastroenterol; 84:1017-1025.
[4] Deyhle P (1980). Results of endoscopic polypectomy in the gastrointestinal tract. Endoscopy; (Suppl): 35-46.
[5] Rex DK, Bond JH, Winawer S, Levin TR, Burt RW, Johnson DA, Kirk LM, Litlin S, Lieberman DA, Waye JD, Church J, Marshall JB, & Riddell RH (2002). Quality in the technical performance of colonoscopy and the continuous quality improvement process for colonoscopy: recommendations of the U.S. Multi-society task force on colorectal cancer. Am J Gastroenterol; 97:1296-1308.
[6] Gmperiale F, Glowinski A, Lin-Cooper N, Rogge D, & Ransohoff F (2008). Five-year risk of colorectal neoplasia after negative screening colonoscopy. N Engl J Med; 359: 1218-1224.
[7] Saniabadi AR, Hanai H, Fukunaga K, Sawada K, Shima C, Bjarnason I, & Lofberg R (2007). Therapeutic leucocytapheresis for inflammatory bowel disease. Transfus Apher Sci; 37:191-200.
[8] Sartor RB (1997). Pathogenesis and immune mechanisms of chronic inflammatory bowel diseases. Am J Gastroenterol; 92 (Suppl): 5S-11S.
[9] Fiocchi C (1998). Inflammatory bowel disease: etiology and pathogenesis. Gastroenterology; 115: 182-205.

[10] Podolsky DK (2002). Inflammatory bowel disease. N Engl J Med; 347: 417-429.
[11] Taffet SL, DAS KM (1983). Sulphasalazine-adverse effects and desensitization. Dig Dis Sci; 28: 833-842.
[12] Present DH (2000). How to do without steroids in inflammatory bowel disease. Inflamm Bowel Dis; 6: 48-57.
[13] Rachmilewitz D (1989). On behalf of an international study group, coated mesalazine (5-aminosalicylic acid) versus sulphasalazine in the treatment of active ulcerative colitis. Br Med J; 298:82-86.
[14] Kornbluth A, Marion JF, Salomon P, Janowitz HD (1995). How effective is current medical therapy for severe ulcerative colitis? J Clin Gastroenterol; 20: 280-284.
[15] Truelove SC, Jewell DP (1974). Intensive intravenous regimens for severe attacks of ulcerative colitis. Lancet; 1:1067-1070.
[16] Jarnerot G, Rolny P, Sandberg-Gertzen H (1985). Intensive intravenous treatment of ulcerative colitis. Gastroenterology; 89: 1005-1013.
[17] Hanauer SB (2004). Medical therapy of ulcerative colitis. Gastroenterology;126: 1582-1592.
[18] O'Keefe SJ (1996). Nutrition and gastrointestinal disease. Scand J Gastroenterol; 220 (Suppl): 52-59.
[19] Kornbluth A, Marion JF, Salomon P, Janowitz HD (1995). How effective is current medical therapy for severe ulcerative colitis? J Clin Gastroenterol; 20: 280-284.
[20] Hyde GM, Thillainayagam AV, Jewell DP (1998). Intravenous cyclosporin as rescue therapy in severe ulcerative colitis: time for a reappraisal? Eur J Gastroenterol Hepatol; 10: 411-413.
[21] Hanauer SB (2001). Can Cyclosporine go it alone in severe ulcerative colitis. Curr Gastroenterol Rep; 3: 455-5-456.
[22] Serkova NJ, Christians U, Benet LZ (2004). Biochemical mechanisms of cyclosporine neurotoxicity. Mol Interv; 4: 97-107.
[23] Tanaka T, Okanobu H, Kuga Y, Yoshifuku Y, Fujino H, Miwata T, Moriya T, Nishida T, Oya T (2010). Clinical and endoscopic features of responders and non-responders to adsorptive leucocytapheresis: a report based on 120 patients with active ulcerative colitis. Gastroenterol Clin Biol;34:687-695.
[24] Saniabadi AR, Hanai H (2010). Therapeutic apheresis from the early civilizations to the twenty-first century. Gastroenterol Clin Biol;34:645-648.
[25] Papadakis KA, Targan SR (200). Role of cytokines in the pathogenesis of inflammatory bowel disease. Annu Rev Med; 51:289-298.
[26] Rutgeerts P, Sandborn WJ, Feagan BG (2005). Infliximab for induction and maintenance therapy for ulcerative colitis. N Engl J Med; 353:2462-2476.
[27] van Dullemen HM, van Deventer SJ, Hommes DW (1995). Treatment of Crohn's disease with anti-tumour necrosis factor chimeric monoclonal antibody (cA2). Gastroenterology; 109: 129-135.
[28] Brown SL, Greene MH, Gershon SK (2002). Tumor necrosis factor antagonist therapy and lymphoma development: twenty-six cases reported to the Food and Drug Administration. Arthritis Rheum; 46: 3151-3158.
[29] Atzeni A, Ardizzone S, Sarzi-Puttini P (2005). Autoantibody profile during short-term infliximab treatment for Crohn's disease: a prospective cohort study. Aliment Pharmacol Ther;22: 453-461.

[30] McCarthy DA, Rampton DS, Liu Y-C (1991). Peripheral blood neutrophils in inflammatory bowel disease: morphological evidence of in vivo activation in active disease. Clin Exp Immunol; 86: 489-493.
[31] Heimann TM, Aufses AH Jr (1985). The role of peripheral lymphocytes in the prediction of recurrence in Crohn's disease. Surg Gynecol Obstet; 160: 295-298.
[32] Suzuki Y, Yoshimura N, Saniabadi AR, Saito Y (2004). Selective neutrophil and monocyte adsorptive apheresis as a first line treatment for steroid naïve patients with active ulcerative colitis: a prospective uncontrolled study. Dig Dis Sci; 49:565-571.
[33] Aoki H, Nakamura K, Suzuki Y (2007). Adacolumn selective leukocyte adsorption apheresis in patients with active ulcerative colitis: clinical efficacy, effects on plasma IL-8 and the expression of toll like receptor 2 on granulocytes. Dig Dis Sci;52:1427-1433.
[34] Tanaka T, Okanobu H, Murakami E (2008). In patients with ulcerative colitis, adsorptive depletion of granulocytes and monocytes impacts mucosal level of neutrophils and clinically is most effective in steroid naive patients, Dig Liver Dis; 40:731-736.
[35] Tibble JA, Sigthorsson G, Bridger D, Fagerhol MK, Bjarnason I (2000). Surrogate markers of intestinal inflammation are predictive of relapse in patients with inflammatory bowel disease. Gastroenterology; 119:15-22.
[36] Schreiber S, Nikolaus S, Hampe J (1999). Tumour necrosis factor alpha and interleukin 1beta in relapse of Crohn's disease. Lancet; 353: 459-461.
[37] Brannigan AE, O'Connell PR, Hurley H (2000). Neutrophil apoptosis is delayed in patients with inflammatory bowel disease. Shock; 13: 361-366.
[38] Lee, A, Whyte M, Haslett C (1993). Inhibition of apoptosis and prolongation of neutrophil functional longevity by inflammatory mediators. J Leukoc Biol; 54:283-288.
[39] Meagher LC, Cousin JM, Seckl JR, Haslett C (1996). Opposing effects of glucocorticoids on the rate of appoptosis in neutrophilic and eosinophilic granulocytes. J Immunol;156: 4422-4428.
[40] Belge KU, Ziegler-Heitbrock HW (2002). The proinflammatory CD14+CD16+ monocytes are a major source of TNF. J Immunol;168:3536-3542.
[41] Hanai H, Iida T, Takeuchi K (2008). Adsorptive depletion of elevated proinflammatory $CD14^{+}CD16^{+}DR^{++}$ monocytes in patients with inflammatory bowel disease. Am J Gastroenterol; 103:1210-1216.
[42] Cohen RD (2005). Treating ulcerative colitis without medications – "Look Mom, No Drugs!" Gastroenterology; 128: 235-236.
[43] Sands BE, Sandborn WJ, Feagan B (2008). A randomized, double-blind, sham-controlled study of granulocyte/monocyte apheresis for active ulcerative colitis. Gastroenterology;135:400-409.
[44] Powrie F, Read S, Mottet C, Uhlig H, Maloy K (2003). Control of immune pathology by regulatory T cells. Novartis Found Symp; 252:92-98.
[45] Maul J, Loddenkemper C, Mundt P, Duchmann R (2005). Peripheral and intestinal regulatory CD4+CD25(high) T cells in inflammatory bowel disease. Gastroenterology;128:1868-1878.

[46] Uhlig HH, Powrie F (2005). The role of mucosal T lymphocytes in regulating intestinal inflammation. Immunopathol; 27:167-180.

[47] Liu H, Hu B, Xu D, Liew FY (2003). CD4+CD25+ regulatory T cells cure murine colitis: the role of IL-10, TGF-beta, and CTLA4. J Immunol; 171:5012-5017.

[48] Huber S, Schramm C, Lehr HA, Blessing M (2004). Cutting edge: TGF-beta signaling is required for the in vivo expansion and immunosuppressive capacity of regulatory CD4+CD25+ T cells. J Immunol;173:6526-6531.

[49] Yokoyama Y, Fukunaga K, Fukuda Y, Matsumoto T (2007). Demonstration of Low-Regulatory $CD25^{(High+)}CD4^{(+)}$ and high-pro-inflammatory $CD28^{(-)}CD4^{(+)}$ T-cell subsets in patients with ulcerative colitis: modified by selective granulocyte and monocyte adsorption apheresis. Dig Dis Sci; 52:2725–2731.

[50] Saniabadi AR, Hanai H, Takeuchi K, Bjarnason I, Lofberg R (2003). Adacolumn, an adsorptive carrier based granulocyte and monocyte apheresis device for the treatment of inflammatory and refractory diseases associated with leukocytes. Ther Apher Dial; 7: 48-59.

[51] Saniabadi AR, Hanai H, Sawada K, Bjarnason I, Lofberg R (2005). Adacolumn for selective leukocytapheresis as a non-pharmacological treatment for patients with disorders of the immune system: an adjunct or an alternative to drug therapy? J Clin Apher; 20: 171-184.

[52] D'Arrigo C, Candal-Couto JJ, Greer M, Veale DJ, Woof JM (1993). Human neutrophil Fc receptor-mediated adhesion under flow: a hallow fiber model of intravascular arrest. Clin. Exp. Immunol; 100:173-179.

[53] Hiraishi K, Takeda Y, Saniabadi A, Kashiwagi N, Adachi M (2003). Studies on the mechanisms of leukocyte adhesion to cellulose acetate beads: an in vitro model to assess the efficacy of cellulose acetate carrier-based granulocyte and monocyte adsorptive apheresis. Ther Apher Dial; 7: 334-340.

[54] Hanai H, Takeda Y, Saniabadi AR, Lofberg R (2011). The mode of actions of the Adacolumn therapeutic leucocytapheresis in patients with inflammatory bowel disease: a concise review. Clin Exp Immunol;163:50-58.

[55] Hanai H, Watanabe F, Takeuchi K & Bjarnason I (2003). Leukcocyte adsorptive apheresis for the treatment of active ulcerative colitis: a prospective uncontrolled pilot study. Clin Gastroenterol Hepatol; 1: 28-35.

[56] Suzuki Y, Yoshimura N, Saito Y, Saniabadi A (2006). A retrospective search for predictors of clinical response to selective granulocyte and monocyte apheresis in patients with ulcerative colitis. Dig Dis Sci; 51: 2031-2038.

6

Virtual Colonoscopy: Indications, Techniques, Findings

Mutlu Saglam and Fatih Ors
Department of Radiology, Gulhane Military Medical Academy, Turkey

1. Introduction

Colorectal cancer (CRC) is the second most prevalent type of cancer in Europe. Early detection and removal of CRC or its precursor lesions by population screening can reduce mortality.[1]

An increasingly popular screening test for colorectal cancer is computed tomographic (CT) colonography, also called virtual colonoscopy (VC). It is a powerful technique for population screening of asymtomatic adults. It has potential advantages over conventional colonoscopy (CC) as it is less invasive, less time-consuming and less expensive. Moreover, no sedation is needed.[2] Its main disadvantages to CC are the exposure of individuals to ionizing radiation and the lack of ability to take tissue samples or to remove polyps during the procedure.[2-6]

CT colonography was first described in 1994 as a radiographic technique in which thin-section images of pneumocolon could be reconstructed by sophisticated software into high-resolution 2D- and 3D images.[7,8] Over time, improvements in hardware and software have allowed faster scanning, reduced exposure to radiation, and better imaging. Newer modes of imaging (called fly-through) can produce results that resemble endoscopic images and permit sophisticated characterization of detected lesions.[7,9-11]

The ability of VC to detect colorectal polyps has been tested in a multitude of studies. VC appeared to be promising in high risk populations, with a reported sensitivity greater than 90% for polyps ≥10 mm. [12-14] To achieve such results, adequate bowel cleaning or fecal tagging and reader experience are essential.

This chapter summarizes the main indications, the current techniques in patient preparation, data acquisition and data analysis as well as imaging features for common benign and malignant colorectal lesions.

2. Indications

CT colonography is used to examine the colon and rectum, and detect abnormalities such as polyps and cancer. There are several clinical indications for CT colonography. They include evaluation of the colon after an incomplete or unsuccessful CC examination and evaluation of the colon proximal to an obstructing neoplasm.[2,15-19] An incomplete CC examination is defined as a failure to intubate the caecum. Incomplete CC may be the result of poor bowel preparation, redundant colon, and patient intolerance to the procedure, spasm, or colonic obstruction caused by a neoplastic or non-neoplastic stenosis. The CT colonography examination can be performed on the same day directly after CC and without additional bowel preparation.[2,20] In cases of an obstructing cancer (Figure 1), CT colonography offers information about the pre-stenotic colon, local tumor invasion, lymph nodes, and distant metastases.[2,21-23] In this case, IV contrast is helpful to enable a complete stating of the patient.[2,19]

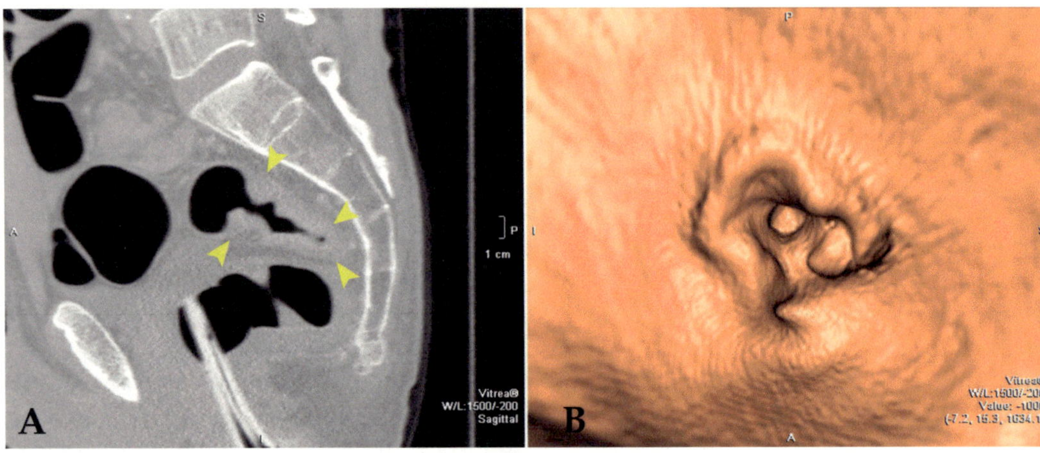

Fig. 1. Incomplete colonoscopy because of a stenotic cancer of the rectum. (A) 2D sagittal CT colonographic image shows circular wall thickening in the rectum (arrowheads). (B) 3D CT colonographic image shows an irregular, circular, stenotic filling defect.

Another indication for CT colonography is the evaluation of patients with contraindications to CC or who refuse other screening options.[2,3] This includes patients in need of anticoagulation, past history of difficult or incomplete colonoscopy, and patients who cannot be sedated due to medical conditions. Furthermore, in cases of advanced patient age, and in frail or immobile patients, CT colonography can be safely performed to exclude neoplastic or stenotic conditions.[2,3,24,25]
At chronic stages of inflammatory bowel disease, CT colonography can provide information on the extent of disease and about stenosis and prestenotic regions, as well as the extracolonic extent and complications of the disease.[2,26-29].

3. Contraindications

Contraindications to CT colonography include acute abdominal pain, recent abdominal or pelvic surgery, abdominal wall hernia with entrapment of colonic loops, and acute inflammatory conditions, such as acute diverticulitis, acute active stage of ulcerative colitis or Crohn's disease, and toxic megacolon. In these conditions, insufflations of the colon can lead to perforation and widespread peritonitis.[2,30-32]. In addition, weight and girth limitations of the scanner, artifacts from metal prosthesis, pregnancy, and patients with claustrophobia are general CT contraindications.[2]

4. CT colonography technique

4.1 Patient preparation

For optimal image quality, the colon should be clean, dry, and completely distended. Residual stool and fluid may lead to a false-negative or false positive diagnosis. A well-prepared colon will facilitate lesion detection and minimize false-positive findings, whereas residual matter in the lumen (e.g., stool, fluid) may stimulate or obscure colonic lesions.[2,12]

There are three commercially available bowel preparations; these include cathartics such as magnesium citrate (LoSo Preparation, EZ-Em Inc, Westbury, NY, USA) and phosphosoda (Fleet Pharmaceuticals, Lynchburg, VA, USA) and colonic lavage solutions such as polyethylene glycol (PEG). Magnesium citrate and phosphosoda are adequate for CT colonography.[2] The polyethylene glycol preparation frequently leaves a large amount of residual fluid in the colon.[3,33] While this preparation is adequate for CC, large amounts of residual fluid will limit CT colonography. At CC, residual fluid can be endoscopically aspirated from the colon. With CT colonography, the examination is typically limited to only two acquisitions (which are supine and prone). While supine and prone imaging allow for fluid redistribution, this does not ensure full mucosal evaluation if a large amount of fluid is present. Thus, for CT colonography, the preparation that provides the least amount of residual fluid will theoretically allow the evaluation of the entire mucosal surface.[2,3]

Phosposoda is contraindicated in patients with known renal failure, preexisting electrolyte abnormalities, congestive heart failure, ascites, or ileus. [2,34] In these circumstances, PEG can be used as an alternative, as it does not result in fluid shifts and electrolyte imbalances. [3,35]

The Fleet Kit consists of a clear fluid diet the day before the examination, as well as a single 45-mL dose of phosphosoda and four bisacodyl tablets the day before the examination. In addition, patients receive a bisacodyl suppository the morning of the examination. The LoSo preparation consists of magnesium citrate and four bisacodyl tablets the day before the examination and a bisacodyl suppository the morning of the examination.[3]

The addition of oral contrast agents will tag residual stool or fluid (Figure 2). Oral contrast agents for stool and fluid tagging consist of meglumine diatrizoate (Gastrografin, Schering AG, Berlin, Germany) and a barium sulfate suspension (Tagitol, E-Z-EM, Lake Success, NY, USA).[6]

The resulting higher attenuation of fecal and fluid residues simplifies their distinction from colonic abnormality. Whereas some authors prefer tagging with barium only, others have reported good results with iodine or a combination of both to achieve fecal and fluid tagging.[2,36-38]

4.2 Bowel distention

Optimal colonic distention is a fundamental prerequisite for CT colonography data evaluation that allows intraluminal evaluation of the large bowel. Underdistended or collapsed segments may hide intraluminal lesions.[2]

Immediately before data acquisition, the patient should evacuate any residual fluid from the rectum. For colonic insufflations, either room air or carbon dioxide (CO_2) can be used. The easiest and cheapest method is manual room air distention via a handheld plastic bulb insufflators. Proponents of CO_2 use argue that its readily absorbance from the colon causes less cramping after the procedure than does room air insufflations. [3,39] Bowel distention is performed in the left decubitus or supine position with a thin, flexible rubber catheter placed in the rectum (e.g., thin plastic or rubber 14F rectal tube, small gauge Foley catheter).[2,40] During the gas insufflation, gentle insufflation is continuous until the patient feels uncomfortable or bloated. Patients are encouraged to keep the gas (room air or CO_2) in as much as possible. The patient is asked to let the technologist know when they begin to feel uncomfortable. Generally this signals that the colon is well distended. If the ileocecal section is incompetent, more gas will be required for optimal distention.[2,3]

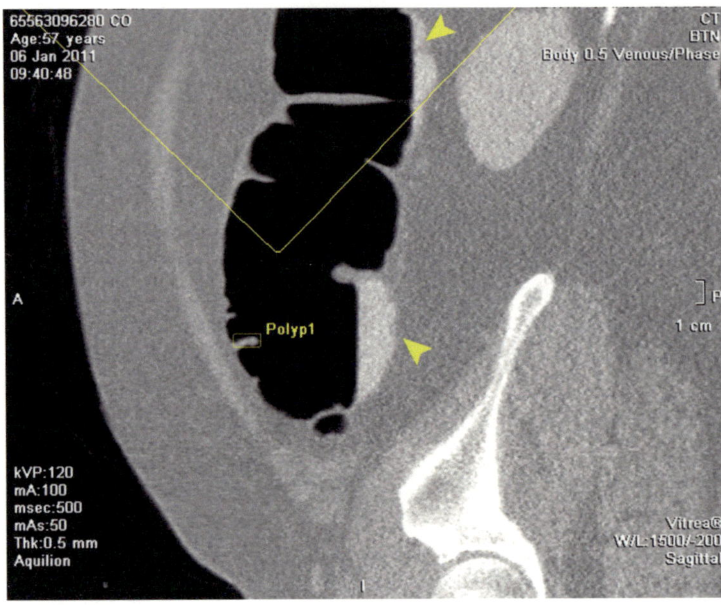

Fig. 2. Fecal tagging with orally ingested barium: 2D sagittal CT colonographic image shows high attenuation of contrast marked fecal residuals and residual fluid (arrowheads), as well as a polyp in the ascending colon.

CO_2 can be administered either manually, over a standard enema bag filled with approximately 3L of gas (via a gas cylinder) attached to a rectal catheter over a connecting tube, or automatically, using a dedicated insufflations device (Protocol colon insufflations system, EZ-Em Inc., Wesbury, NY, USA). This device electronically controls the flow rate of CO_2, the total administered gas volume, and the intracolonic pressure (which is limited up to a maximum of 25 mmHg).[2,41,42] This generally will take 2-4L of gas, depending on the patient's individual colonic anatomy.[2]

After distention, the catheter is left in the rectum, and a single scout CT image is obtained with the patient in the supine position to verify adequate bowel distention (Figure 3). If adequate bowel distention is present, the CT examination is performed. Otherwise, additional gas is insufflated into the rectum, according to the scout image. Following the supine axial image acquisition, the patient is turned to the prone position. Several additional puffs of air are then administered, or CO_2 is continuously administered. After a second scout localizing image is obtained, the process is repeated over the same z-axis range. Supine and prone imaging doubles the radiation dose but is essential to allow optimal bowel distention, redistribution of residual fluid, and differentiation of fecal material from polyps because visualization of mobility of a filling defect implies residual fecal material.[3] Before prone image acquisition, another scout scan is obtained with additional gaseous insufflation if needed.[2,3]

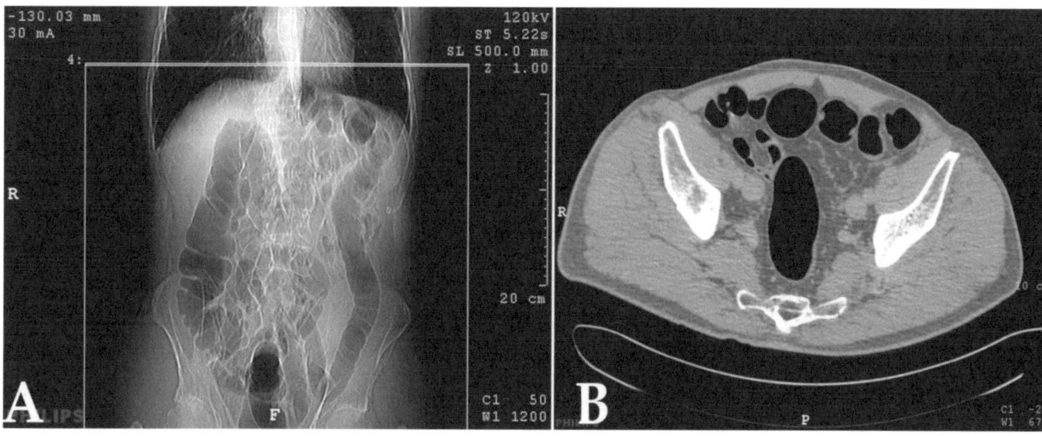

Fig. 3. (A) Supine scout CT image and (B) 2D transverse CT colonographic image show adequate distension of colonic segments, allowing diagnostic examination.

The i.v. administration of antispasmotic agents (buscopan, or glucagon) may improve colonic distention and reduce spasms. The general opinion is that IV spasmolytics should not be administered routinely, but can be used if patients experience pain, discomfort, or spasm.[2,43]
Bowel distention may lead to perforation of the bowel in rare cases. In most of the reported cases, perforation occurred in symptomatic patients with acute inflammatory or stenotic colons.[2,30-32]

4.3 Data acquisition

CT scanning is ideally performed on a multi-detector computed tomography (MDCT) scanner in both the supine and the prone positions with a thin collimation. MDCT has several technical advantages over single-detector CT, including faster imaging times, reduced exposure to radiation and acquisition of multiple thin sections with nearly isotropic voxels.[2,3,7,11,22,23,43-46] Moreover, motion artifacts from respiration and peristalsis are decreased or eliminated with MDCT.[3]
Thin sections are a prerequisite for high-quality multiplanar reformations (MPR) and 3D reconstructions. Near-isotropic imaging is already provided on a 4-row MDCT scanner with a detector configuration of 4 mm x 1 mm (minimal slice thickness of 1.25 mm), which allows scanning of abdomen during a 30-s breath-hold. With a 16-row or 64-row MDCT scanner, and a detector configuration of 16 mm x 0.75 mm or 64 mm x 0.6 mm, scanning is completed in 11-12 s or 6-7 s. Such datasets can be reconstructed as 1 mm sections overlapped every 0.7 mm.[2]
One of the major limitations of CT colonography is the relatively high radiation exposure, and thus, increasing attention has been focused on low-dose protocols. Because a thin collimation is necessary for CT colonography, dose reduction is widely achieved by

reducing the miliampere-seconds level. Generally useful exposure settings are 120kVp and 50-100mAs in the prone and in supine positions.[2] Use of automated dose modulation techniques that adapt mAs values to patient anatomy should always be used, if these techniques are available on the CT scanner.[2,47]

4.4 Data analysis

Image processing and interpretation is performed on a commercially available computer workstation equipped with dedicated CT colonography software. In addition to 2D axial and MPR in a cine mode, such systems provide an interactive, manual, mouse-driven, automated or semi-automated, virtual "fly-trough" of the surface- or volume-rendered 3D intraluminal images.[2]
There are two primary techniques for data interpretation: a primary 2D or a primary 3D approach (Figure 4). The combined use of both, 2D and 3D visualization techniques has been shown to be superior to the evaluation of single 3D or 2D views, with regard to sensitivity and specificity.[2,48,49]

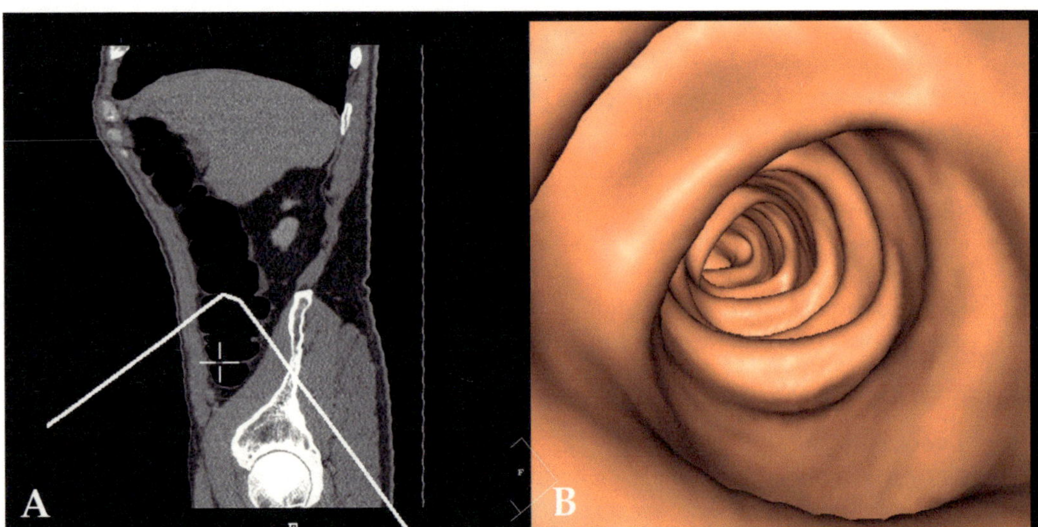

Fig. 4. (A) 2D sagittal CT colonographic image and (B) 3D CT colonographic image show a normal smooth colonic wall.

With a primary 2D technique, the entire colon is evaluated by using the transverse source images. This is accomplished at a specialized workstation, and the colon is "tracked" from the rectum to the cecum by using the supine images. This is facilitated by cine scrolling of images through the entire colon. If an abnormality is detected; coronal, sagittal, and endoluminal reformatted images are used to help determine whether the abnormality is a polyp, fold, or fecal matter.[3] Primary 2D evaluation provides information about the attenuation of findings during the search process and is more time-efficient.[2,48,50]
Primary 3D evaluation is based on 3D virtual endoscopy in an antegrade and retrograde fashion. Primary 3D evaluation was shown to be sensitive for polyp detection because both, the conspicuity, especially of small and medium-sized polyps, and the duration of visualization, are increased.[2,38] The primary 3D evaluation is time-consuming because it

must be performed in antegrade and retrograde fashion for the perception of lesions behind haustral folds. Collapsed segments must be evaluated alternatively, by 2D planar images.[2]
There are several limitations of the primary 3D evaluation. First, there are blind spots in the colon when 3D endoluminal views are used.[3,51] Several workstations currently have the capacity to display these blind areas to the reviewer after the 3D navigation is performed, which should allow a more complete visualization of the colon when a primary 3D interpretation technique is used. These are virtual dissection, panaromic, unfolded cube projection, and translucency rendering.[2,3,51] A second limitation of 3D endoluminal fly-through imaging is that the centerline cannot be generated when segments of the colon are not well distended. Third, in over-distended segments the centerline may jump to an adjacent distended loop.[3]
In addition to polyp size, segmental location, morphologic type (pedunculated, sessile, or flat), and diagnostic confidence score are recorded for each polyp.[52] For a number of reasons, the presence of diminutive lesions should not be mentioned. Tiny polyps are not clinically relevant, yet mentioning them can cause undue anxiety in patients and referring physicians.[38,52-54] Most diminutive "lesions" detected at CT colonography cannot be found at subsequent CC, representing either false-positive CT colonography findings or false-negative CC findings.[52]
There are three criteria to use with 2D and 3D imaging that help distinguish residual fecal material from polyps. First, the presence of internal gas or areas of high attenuation suggest that a lesion is residual fecal material, since colorectal polyps are homogeneous in attenuation.[3,55,56] The second criterion is morphology. Morphologically, polyps and small cancers have rounded or lobulated smooth borders. Residual fecal material may have a similar morphology. However, if a lesion shows geometric or irregularly angled borders, it almost always represents residual fecal material.[3,50] Mobility of a lesion is the third criterion. Stool tends to move to the dependent surface of the colonic mucosa when a patient is turned from the supine to the prone position.[3,56,57] Polyps maintain their position with respect to the bowel surface (ventral or dorsal) regardless of the patient's position. However, caution is required since pedunculated polyps and sessile polyps in segments of the colon with a long mesentery appear to be mobile.[3,58]
Computer-aided detection (CAD) systems are software programs that automatically highlight polyp "candidates" and thus support the radiologist by pointing out possible abnormalities that may otherwise have been missed. Based on morphologic and attenuation characteristics, the reader then decides whether the "candidate lesion" is a true- or a false-positive finding. Recent CAD algorithms showed a promising performance, with a reported a CAD sensitivity of 89,3% for adenomas ≥10 mm.[2,59]

5. Findings

One of the most common findings detected with CT colonography is diverticular disease. On 2D CT colonography images (Figure 5A), diverticula appear as air-filled outpouchings of the colonic wall. On the 3D virtual endoscopic images (Figure 5B), the diverticular orifice can be recognized as a complete dark ring.[2,60]
Polyps are the most common benign lesions of the colon. The risk of malignant transformation increases with the size of the polyp. On 2D plane images (Figure 6A and 6C), polyps have homogenous, soft tissue attenuation. On 3D virtual endoscopic images (Figure 6B and 6D), polypoid lesions present as a sessile or stalked, round, oval, or lobulated

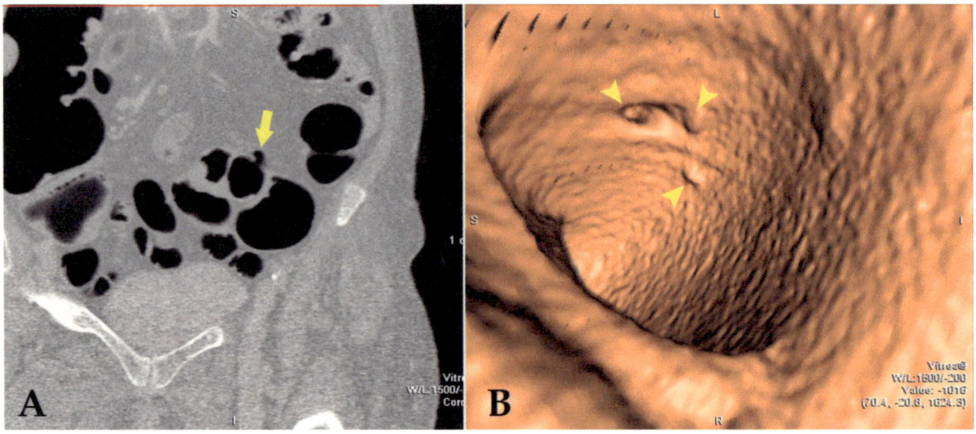

Fig. 5. The appearance of diverticula on (A) the 2D axial CT colonographic image (arrow) and (B) the 3D CT colonographic image (arrowheads).

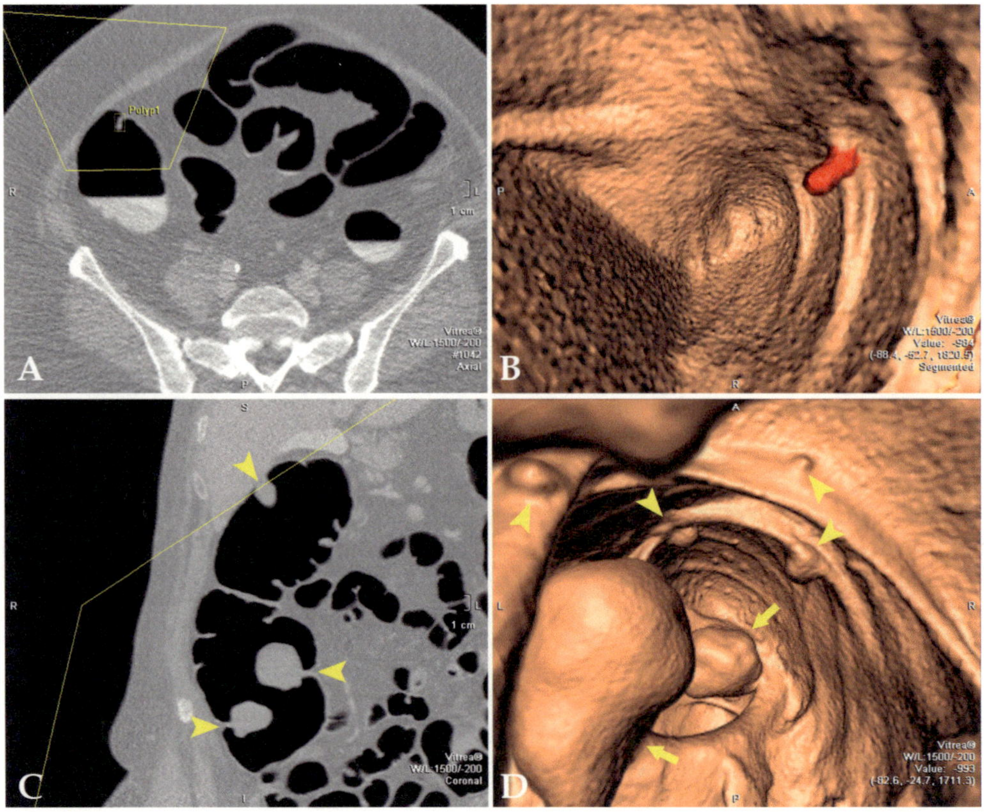

Fig. 6. (A) The appearance of a stalked polyp of the assending colon on 2D axial CT colonographic image. (B) Translucency rendering view shows a homogenous red bulging revealing the polyp. (C) The appearance of stalked polyps on 2D coronal CT colonographic image (arrowheads). (D) 3D CT colonographic image shows stalked (arrows) and sessile (arrowheads) polyps.

intraluminal filling defect. Typically, the margin to the normal mucosa is displayed as an incomplete ring shadow.[2,61] Flat polyps are defined as lesions with a height less than 50% of the lesion width. In CT colonography, flat polyps appear as a fairly circumscribed area of mild wall thickening with homogenous soft tissue attenuation. Sometimes a mild nodularity is found on the surface by 3D endoluminal images.[2,62]

Lipomas are the most common submucosal lesions in the colon (especially common on the ileocecal valve). On 2D plane images, lipomas are present as homogenous fatty lesions. On 3D virtual endoscopic images, lipomas are present as a sessile or pedunculated polpoid intraluminal filling defect, most often with a smooth surface. In general, small lipomas need no further treatment; only large lipomas require endoscopic resection because they can lead to intusseption.[2,61]

Colorectal cancer is the most common colonic primary tumour. Colorectal cancer(Figure 7) typically shows extensive focal polypoid, asymmetric, or circular wall thickening with short extension (<5cm), especially with shoulder formation.[2,60,63] Pericolonic lymph nodes and distant metastases are signs of progression of the disease and can be evaluated using 2D axial source images and MPR views.[2]

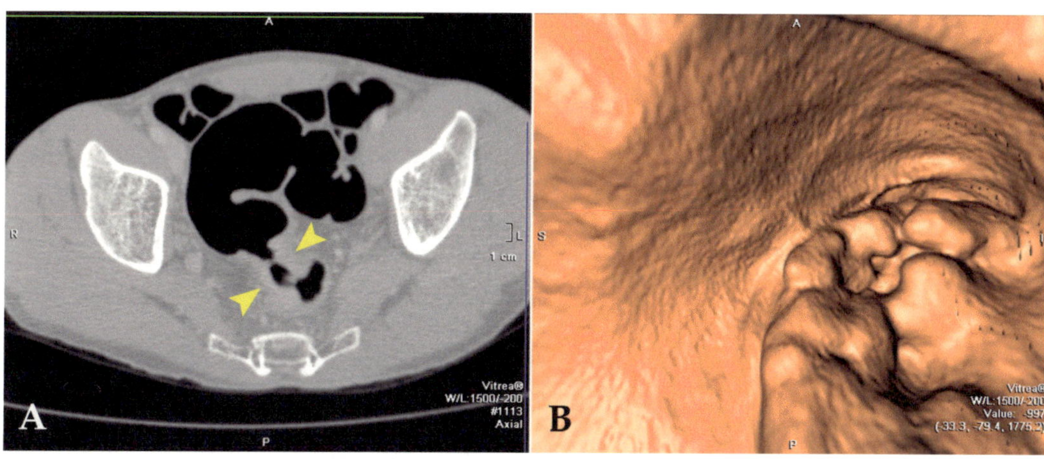

Fig. 7. (A) 2D axial CT colonographic image shows circular wall thickening in the rectum (arrowheads). (B) 3D CT colonographic image shows an irregular, circular, stenotic filling defect.

6. Pitfalls

CT colonography has a number of potential pitfalls. Some pitfalls, such as prominent and complex folds, diverticular fold thickening, and shifting of pedunculated polyps, present more of a problem at 2D evaluation. Other pitfalls, such as annular masses, submucosal or extrinsic lesions, and impacted diverticula, are more an issue at 3D evaluation. With a biphasic interpretive approach, most pitfalls are easily recognized because of the complementary nature of the 2D and 3D displays.[52]

7. Conclusion

CT colonography is highly sensitive for colorectal cancer, especially when both cathartic and tagging agents are combined in the bowel preparation. Given the relatively low prevalence of colorectal cancer, primary CT colonography may be more suitable than CC for initial investigation of suspected colorectal cancer.

8. References

[1] De Wijkerslooth TR, de Haan MC, Stoop EM, Deutekom M, Fockens P, Bossuyt PM, Thomeer M, van Ballegooijen M, Essink-Bot ML, van Leerdam, ME, Kuipers EJ, Dekker E, Stoker J. Study protocol: population screening for colorectal cancer by colonoscopy or CT colonography: a randomized controlled trial. BMC Gastroenterol 2010; 10:47.

[2] Mang T, Graser A, Schima W, Maier A. CT colonography: techniques, indications, findings. EJR 2007; 61:388-99.

[3] Macari M, Bini EJ. CT colonography: where have we been and where are we going? Radiology 2005; 237:819-33.

[4] Silva AC, Hara AK, Leighton JA, Heppell JP. CT colonography with intravenous contrast material: varied appearances of colo-rectal carcinoma. Radiographics 2005; 25(5):1321-34.

[5] Svensson MH, Svensson E, Lasson A, Hellstrom M. Patient acceptance of CT colonography and conventional colonoscopy; prospective comparative study in patients with or suspected of having colorectal disease. Radiology 2002; 222:337-45.

[6] Silva AC, Vens EA, Hara AK, Fletcher JG, Fidler JL, Johnson CD. Evaluation of benign and malignant rectal lesions with CT colonography and endoscopic correlation. Radiographics 2006; 26(4):1085-99.

[7] Mulhall BP, Veerappan GR, Jackson Jeffrey. Meta-analysisi: computed tomographic colonography. Annals of Internal Medicine 2005; 142(8):635-50.

[8] Vining DJ, Gelfand DW, Bechtold RE, Scharling ES, Grishaw EK, Shifrin GY. Technical feasibility of colon imaging with helical CT and virtual reality (Abstract). Am J Roentgenol 1994; 162 (Suppl):S104.

[9] Geenen RW, Hussain SM, Cademartiri F, Poley JW, Siersema PD, Shifrin GP. CT and MR colonography: scanning techniques, postprocessing, and emphasis on polyp detection. Radiograğhics 2004; 24:e18.

[10] Dachman AH, Yoshida H. Virtual colonoscopy; past, present, and future. Radiol Clin North Am 2003; 41:377-93.

[11] Laghi A, Lannaccone R, Panebianco V, Carbone L, Passariello R. Multislice CT colonography: technical developments. Semin Ultrasound CT MR. 2001; 22: 425-31.

[12] Mang T, Maier A, Plank C, Mueller-Mang C, Herold C, Schima W. Pitfalls in multi-detector row CT colonography: a systematic approach. Radiographics 2007; 27:431-54.

[13] Pickhardt PJ, Hassan C, Halligan S, Marmo R. Colorectal Cancer: CT Colonography and colonoscopy for detection--systematic rewiev and meta-analysis (Abstract). Radiology 2011 Mar 17 [Epub ahead of print].

[14] Filippone A, Ambrosini R, Fuschi M, Marinelli T, Genovesi D, Bonomo L. Preoperative T and N staging of colorectal cancer: accuracy of contrast-enhanced multi-detector row CT colonography-initial experience. Radiology 2004; 231: 83-90.

[15] Fenlon HM, McAneny DB, Nunes DP, Clarke PD, Ferrucci JT. Occlusive colon carcinoma: virtual colonoscopy in the preoperative evaluation of the proximal colon. Radiology 1999; 210:423-28.

[16] Macari M, Berman P, Dicker M, Milano A, Megibow AJ. Usefulness of CT colonography in patients with incomplete colonoscopy. AJR Am J Roentgenol 1999: 173:561-64.

[17] Morrin MM, Farrell RJ, Raptopoulos V, MacGee JB, Bleday R, Kruskal JB. Role of virtual computed tomographic colonography in patients with colorectal cancers and obstructing colorectal lesions. Dis Colon Rectum 2000; 43:303-11.

[18] Morrin MM, Kruskal JB, Farrell RJ, Goldberg SN, McGee JB, Raptopoulos V. Endoluminal CT colonography after an incomplete endoscopic colonoscopy. AJR Am J Roentgenol 1999; 172: 913-18.

[19] Neri E, Giusti P, Battolla L, Vagli P, Boraschi, R, Caramella D, Bartolozzi C. Colorectal cancer: role of CT colonography in preoperative evaluation after incomplete colonoscopy. Radiology 2002; 223:615-19.

[20] Laghi A. Virtual colonoscopy: clinical application. Eur Radiol 2005; 15 (Suppl 4):D138-41.

[21] Chung DJ, Huh KC, Choi WJ, Kim JK. CT colonography using 16-MDCT in the evaluation of colorectal cancer. AJR Am J Roentgenol 2005; 184:98-103.

[22] Filippone A, Ambrosini R, Fuschi M, Marinelli T, Genovesi D, Bonomo L. Preoperative T and N staging of colorectal cancer: accuracy of contrast-enhanced multi-detector row CT colonography-initial experience. Radiology 2004; 231: 83-90.

[23] Iannacone R, Laghi A, Passariello R. Colorectal carcinoma: detection and staging with multislice CT (MSCT) colonography. Abdom Imaging 2005; 30:13-19.

[24] Fletcher JG, Johnson CD, Krueger WR, Ahlquist DA, Nelson H, Ilstrup D, Harmsen WS, Corcoran KE. Contrast-enhanced CT colonography in recurrent colorectal carcinoma: feasibility of simultaneous evaluation of metastatic disease, local recurrence, and metachronous neoplasia in colorectal carcinoma. AJR Am J Roentgenol 2002; 178(2):283-90.

[25] Laghi A, Iannaccone R, Bria E, Carbone I, Trasatti L, Piacentini F, Lauro S, Vecchione A, Passariello R. Contrast-enhanced computed tomographic colonography in the follow-up colorectal cancer patients: a feasibility study. Eur Radiol 2003; 13(4):883-9.

[26] Biacone L, Fiori R, Tosti C, Marinetti A, Catarinacci M, De Nigris F, Simonetti G, Pallone F. Vitual colonoscopy compared with conventional colonoscopy for structuring postoperative recurrence in Crohn`s disease. Inflamm Bowel Dis 2003; 9(6):343-50.

[27] Tarjan Z, Zagoni T, Gyorke T, Mester A, Karlinger K, Mako EK. Spiral CT colonography in imflammatory bowel disease. Eur J Radiol 2000; 35:193-8.

[28] Ota Y, Matsui T, Ono H, Uno H, Matake H, Tsuda S, Sakurai T, Yao T. Value of virtual computed tomographic colonography for Crohn`s colitis: comparison with endoscopy and barium enema. Abdom Imaging 2003; 28:778-83.

[29] Saglam M, Ors F, Nikola S, Yildirim D, Tasar M, Tuzun A, Bozlar U. Sonographic and multidetector computed tomographic findings of 6 cases with inflammatory bowel disease. Gulhane Med J 2007; 49:129-31.

[30] Burling D, Halligan S, Slater A, Noakes MJ, Taylor SA. Potentially serious adverse events at CT colonography in symptomatic patients: national survey of the United Kingdom. Radiology 2006; 239:464-41.

[31] Pickhardt PJ. Incidence colonic perforation at CT colonography: review of exiting data and implications for screening of asymptomatic adults. Radiology 2006; 239:313-6.

[32] Sosna J, Blachar A, Amitai M, Barmeir E, Peled N, Goldberg SN, Bar-Ziv J. Colonic perforation at CT colonography: assessment of risk in a multicenter large cohort. 2006; 239(2):457-63.

[33] Macari M, Pedrosa I, Lavelle M, Milano A, Dicker M, Megibow AJ, Xue X. Effect of different bowel preparations on residual fluid at CT colonography. Radiology 2001;218(1):274-7

[34] Fass R, Do S, Hixson LJ. Fatal hyperphosphatemia following Fleet Phospo-Soda in apatient with colonic ileus. Am J Gastroenterol 1993; 88:929-32.

[35] Macari M, Bini EJ, Jacobs SL, Lui YW, Laks S, Milano A, Babb J. Clinical significance of missed polyps at CT colonography. AJR Am J Roentgenol 2004; 183(1):127-34.

[36] Lefere PA, Gryspeerdt SS, Dewyspelaere J, Baekelandt M, Van Holsbeeck BG. Dietary fecal tagging as a cleansing method before CT colonography: initial results polyp detection and patient acceptance. Radiology 2002; 224:393-403.

[37] Iannaccone R, Laghi A, Cataalano C, Mangiapane F, Lamazza A, Schillaci A, Sinibaldi G, Murakami T, Sammartino P, Hori M, Piacentini F, Nofroni I, Stipa V, Passariello R. Computed tomographic colonography without cathartic preparation for the detection of colorectal polyps. Gastroenterology 2004; 127(5):1300-11.

[38] Pickhardt PJ, Choi JR, Hwang I, Schindler WR. Computed tomographic virtual colonoscopy to screen for colorectal neoplasia in asymptomatic adults. N Eng J Med 2003; 349(23):2191-200.

[39] Stevenson GW, Wilson JA, Wilkinson J, Norman G, Goodacre RL. Pain following colonoscopy: elimination with carbon dioxide. Gastrointest Endosc 1992; 38:564-7.

[40] Dachman AH. Advice for optimizing colonic distention and minizing risk of perforation during CT colonography. Radiology 2006; 239:317-21.

[41] Burling D, Taylor SA, Halligan S, Gartner L, Paliwalla M, Peiris C, Singh L, Bassett P, Bartram C. Automated insufflations of carbon dioxide for MDCT colonography: distention and patient experience compared with manual insufflations. AJR Am J Roentgenol 2006; 186(1):96-103.

[42] Shinners TJ, Pickhardt PJ, Taylor AJ, Jones DA, Olsen CH. Patient-controlled room air insufflations versus automated carbon dioxide delivery for CT colonography. AJR Am J Roentgenol 2006; 186:1491-6.

[43] Rogalla P, Meiri N, Ruckert JC, Hamm B. Colonography using multislice CT Eur J Radiol 2000; 36:81-5.

[44] Wessling J, Fischbach R, Meier N, Allkemper T, Klusmeier J, Ludwig K, Heindel W. CT colonography: protocol optimization with multi-detector row CT-study in an anthropomorphic colon phantom. Radiology 2003; 228(3):753-9.

[45] Taylor SA, Halligan S, Bartram CI, Morgan PR, Talbot IC, Fry N, Saunders BP, Khosraviani K, Atkin W.Multi-detector row CT colonography: effect of collimation, pitch, and orientation on polyp detection in a human colectomy specimen. Radiology 2003; 229(2):109-18.
[46] Taylor Sa, Halligan S, Saunders BP, Morley S, Riesewyk C, Atkin W, Bartram CI. Use of multidetector-row CT colonography for detection of colorectal neoplasia in patients referred via the department of health "2-week-wait" initiative. Clin Radiol 2003; 58(11):855-61.
[47] Craser A, Wintersperger BJ, Suess C, Reiser MF, Becker CR. Dose reduction and image quality in MDCT colonography using the current modulation. AJR Am J Roentgenol 2006; 187:695-701.
[48] Dachman AH, Kuniyoshi JK, Boyle CM, Samara Y, Hoffmann KR, Rubin DT, Hanan I. CT colonography with three-dimensional problem solving for detection of colonic polyps. AJR Am J Roentgenol 1998; 171(4):989-95.
[49] Royster AP, Fenlon HM, Clarke PD, Nunes DP, Ferruci JT. CT colonoscopy of colorectal neoplasms: two—dimensional and three-dimensional virtual-reality techniques with colonoscopic correlation. AJR Am J Roentgenol 1998; 169:1237-42.
[50] Macari M, Milano A, Lavelle M, Berman P, Megibow AJ. Comparison of time-efficient CT colonography with two-three-dimensional colonic evaluation for detecting colorectal polyps. AJR Am J Roentgenol 2000; 174:1543-9.
[51] Beaulieu Cf, Jeffrey RB, Karadi C, Paik DS, Napel S. Display modes for CT colonography. II. Blinded comparison of axial CT and virtual endoscopic and panoramic endoscopic volume-rendered studies. Radiology 1999; 212(1):203-12.
[52] Pickhardt PJ. Screening CT colonography: how I do it. AJR Am J Roentgenol 2007; 189:290-8.
[53] Zalis ME, Barish MA, Choi JR, Dachman AH, Fenlon HM, Ferrucci JT, Glick SN, Laghi A, Macari M, McFarland EG, Morrin MM, Pickhardt PJ, Soto J, Yee J. CT colonography reporting and data system: a consensus proposal. Radiology 2005; 236(1):3-9.
[54] Pickhardt PJ. CT colonography (virtual colonoscopy) for primary colorectal screening: challenges facing clinical implementation. Abdom Imaging 2005; 30:1-4.
[55] Macari M, Megibow AJ. Pitfalls of using three dimensional CT colonography with two dimensional imaging correlation. AJR Am J Roentgenol 2001; 176:137-43.
[56] Fletcher JG, Johnson CD, MacCarty RL, Welch TJ, Reed JE, Hara AK. CT colonography: potential pitfalls and problem solving techniques. AJR Am J Roentgenol 1999; 172:1271-8.
[57] Yee J, Kumar NN, Hung RK, Akekar GA, Kumar PR, Wall SD. Comparison of supine and prone scanning separately and in combination at CT colonography. Radiology 2003; 226(3):653-61.
[58] Laks S, Macari M, Bini EJ. Positional change in colon polyps at CT colonography. Radiology 2004; 231(3):761-6.
[59] Summers RM, Yao J, Pickhardt PJ, Franaszek M, Bitter I, Brickman D, Krishna V, Choi JR. Computed tomographic virtual colonoscopy computer-aided polyp detection in a screening population. Gastroenterology 2005; 129:1832-44.

[60] Fenlon HM, Clarke PD, Ferrucci JT. Virtual colonoscopy: imaging features with colonoscopic correlation. AJR Am J Roentgenol 1998; 170:1303-9.

[61] Macari M, Bini EJ, Jacobs SL, Lange N, Lui YW. Filling defects at CT colonography: pseudo- and diminutive lesions (the good), polyps (the bad), flat lesions, masses, and carcinomas (the ugly). Radiographics 2003; 23:1073-91.

[62] Rembacken BJ, Fujii T, Cairns A, Dixon MF, Yoshida S, Chalmers DM, Axon AT.Flat and depressed colonic neoplasms: a prospective study of 1000 colonoscopies in the UK. Lancet 2000; 355:1211-4.

[63] Taylor SA, Halligan S, Bartram CI. CT colonography: methods, pathology and pitfalls. Clin Radiol 2003; 58:179-90.

7

Emergency Total Intraoperative Enteroscopy Using a Colonoscope

Francisco Pérez-Roldán, Pedro González-Carro and María Concepción Villafáñez-García
Hospital General La Mancha-Centro
Alcázar de San Juan
Spain

1. Introduction

Hemodynamically unstable lower gastrointestinal bleeding is a challenge for on-call teams, especially when symptom severity leaves no time to apply diagnostic techniques. While colonoscopy and gastroduodenoscopy performed before arteriography or scintigraphy are considered the usual diagnostic tools, capsule endoscopy provides new options in patients with stable digestive bleeding that is difficult to locate. Computed tomography (CT) angiography is beginning to replace arteriography and labeled red cell scintigraphy. Nonetheless, the primary objective is to locate the bleeding source, and, in cases where this must be located by surgery, intraoperative enteroscopy using a colonoscopy can be applied. In fact, intraoperative enteroscopy is considered effective from a diagnostic and therapeutic perspective in selected patients, for example, those with severe gastrointestinal bleeding of no apparent etiology and for whom other diagnostic techniques are ineffective or unavailable. This technique ensures that surgical resection is minimally invasive.

2. Etiology of severe gastrointestinal bleeding

Massive gastrointestinal bleeding is often associated with the upper digestive tract. Therefore, in suspected upper gastrointestinal bleeding, the first technique to be applied is esophagogastroduodenoscopy, which makes it possible to diagnose lesions as far as the angle of Treitz. If the patient does not present hematemesis and upper endoscopy findings are normal, the diagnosis is lower gastrointestinal bleeding.

Colonoscopy is one of two tools used to assess lower gastrointestinal bleeding. Some studies have shown that it can identify the bleeding source in slightly more than 70% of patients. Colonoscopy can be performed as an emergency technique or as an elective technique, depending on hemodynamic status, and in many cases it enables us to diagnose and treat a lesion endoscopically. However, in the case of massive bleeding, the effectiveness of colonoscopy could be limited by its poor visibility.

In fact, massive lower gastrointestinal bleeding with an unidentified source is one of the most severe problems faced by a Digestive Service or General Surgery Service. Bleeding of the small intestine is rare, accounting for 2-10% of all cases of gastrointestinal bleeding. The most common causes of gastrointestinal bleeding are vascular malformations (especially angiodysplasia), tumors (including lymphoma), ulcers (caused by nonsteroidal anti-inflammatory drugs, Crohn disease, and enteritis), Meckel diverticulum, diverticulum of the jejunum and ileum, aortoenteric fistula, hemobilia, and pancreatic bleeding (Table 1). Meckel diverticulum should always be taken into consideration in children and young adults. However, in adults and elderly people, the most frequent causes are vascular lesions followed by tumors, irrespective of the presentation of the bleeding.

Upper gastrointestinal tract	Small bowel	Large bowel
Peptic ulcer disease 40-79%	Angiodysplasia 70-80%	Diverticular disease 17-40%
Gastritis/duodenitis 5-30%	Jejunoileal diverticula	Arteriovenous malformations 2-30%
Esophageal varices 6-21%	Meckel diverticulum	Colitis (ischemia, IBD, radiation) 9-21%
Mallory-Weiss tear 3-15%	Benign/malignant neoplasm	Colonic neoplasm 5-8%
Esophagitis 2-8%	Lymphomas	Post-polypectomy bleeding 3-6%
Gastric cancer 2-3%	Enteritis	Anorectal conditions 4-10%
Dieulafoy lesion <1%	Crohn disease	Colonic tuberculosis
Gastric arteriovenous malformation <1%	Aortoduodenal fistula	
Portal gastropathy <1%	Hemobilia, hemosuccus pancreaticus	

Table 1. Causes of acute massive gastrointestinal bleeding.
(IBD, inflammatory bowel disease)

3. Radiologic evaluation of severe gastrointestinal bleeding

In cases of massive lower gastrointestinal bleeding where it is not possible to diagnose the cause, other diagnostic methods should be applied to identify the bleeding source. The primary objective of traditional radiologic tests, including labeled red blood cell scintigraphy and angiography, is localization of the bleeding source so that therapeutic embolization of the feeding vessel can be performed. Novel imaging studies such as CT enterography and CT angiography not only allow localization of the source and diagnosis of the underlying etiology of gastrointestinal bleeding, but also facilitate luminal and extraluminal evaluation of the small bowel.

Mesenteric arteriography is widely used to assess massive gastrointestinal bleeding, although it is also used to assess bleeding of obscure origin that cannot be identified by endoscopy. It is very effective for detecting arteriovenous malformations and tumors—these lesions present a characteristic vascular pattern—and, in active bleeding, it identifies the bleeding source in 50% of patients. It has the added advantage that it can embolize the feeding artery and control bleeding, thus stabilizing the patient. This is particularly important in many high-risk surgical patients, since the technique is safe, morbidity and mortality are low, and ischemia and rebleeding are very uncommon.

Helical CT with intravenous contrast or CT angiography is similar to arteriography, although it could produce false negatives due to the intermittent nature of bleeding. In cases of massive bleeding, diagnostic efficacy (extravasated contrast medium in the intestine during the arterial phase) reaches 88.5%, with a sensitivity of 90.9% and a specificity of 99%. The location of the source of extravasation on the CT angiogram corresponds exactly to the results of arteriography. Once the bleeding source is found, therapeutic angiography can be applied or alternative treatment can be selected depending on the findings.

CT enterography and CT enteroclysis are dedicated examinations of the small bowel that allow the detection of vascular lesions and tumors. The technique optimizes luminal distension by administering larger volumes of neutral oral contrast via peroral (CT enterography) or nasojejunal intubation (CT enteroclysis), thereby allowing optimal visualization of mucosal and vascular detail. The evaluation of gastrointestinal bleeding usually involves multiphasic imaging (arterial, enteric, and delayed imaging, with or without precontrast images). Typical features of angiodysplasia on CT include the presence of a vascular tuft in the arterial phase and an early draining mesenteric vein. Active bleeding may also be identified on multiphasic imaging by the increasing accumulation of contrast in the small bowel lumen. CT enterography has the added advantage being able to identify small bowel strictures/obstruction prior to capsule endoscopy and provides important information on luminal and extraluminal findings that cannot be detected on capsule endoscopy.

Lastly, we must remember other radiologic tests such as *^{99m}Tc red blood cell scintigraphy*, a noninvasive examination that can detect bleeding with a loss lower than that observed with arteriography (0.1-0.4 ml/min). It can identify an indeterminate source in 20-40% of patients—this percentage rises to 68% when there is active bleeding—and is generally used to detect the source of intestinal bleeding and improve the management of patients with active bleeding, thus making it possible to choose the best therapeutic option, which is often arteriography. 99mTc red blood cell scintigraphy is the technique of choice in the diagnosis of Meckel diverticulum. An additional approach in this disease is *technetium 99m pertechnetate scintigraphy (MeckelScan)*, which makes it possible to detect ectopic gastric mucosa with 64-100% sensitivity; however, its main disadvantage is the rapid isotope washout when there is active gastrointestinal bleeding.

4. Endoscopic evaluation of severe gastrointestinal bleeding

In the last few years, several advances have been made in endoscopy techniques applied for the diagnosis and treatment of diseases of the gastrointestinal tract. However, few of these advances are of benefit in diseases of the small bowel, because access with an endoscope remains difficult. Since the introduction of push endoscopy in 1971, only the proximal jejunum could be examined to about 50 cm from the ligament of Treitz. Examination of the small intestine has improved with more recent discoveries, including include capsule endoscopy, double-balloon enteroscopy, and spiral enteroscopy. Capsule endoscopy as a

diagnostic method has revealed a new challenge, namely, determination of the confirmatory and therapeutic approach to the lesions found.
Gastroscopy and colonoscopy are both available in all hospitals. If these techniques do not confirm the diagnosis in patients with massive low gastrointestinal bleeding, we must determine the cause of the lesion and decide how to diagnose and treat it. Bleeding of the small intestine has been a complex diagnostic problem for many years, because this organ could not be explored using endoscopy and the cause of the bleeding was difficult to locate using more conventional techniques. Severe active intestinal bleeding can be diagnosed using radiological techniques (see above) and endoscopic techniques, including push enteroscopy, capsule endoscopy, balloon-assisted enteroscopy, spiral enteroscopy, and endoscopy-assisted laparoscopy-laparotomy (intraoperative enteroscopy). However, these techniques are only available in tertiary hospitals. Secondary hospitals do not usually have all of the techniques described and the distance to the nearest reference hospital must be taken into account. Consequently, it is necessary to act more effectively and invasively in extreme cases (eg, intraoperative enteroscopy). Below, we provide a brief summary of the different endoscopic techniques.
Push enteroscopy. For several years, push enteroscopy has been the most widely used and effective diagnostic procedure for direct evaluation of the intestinal mucosa. One of its limitations is that only the proximal jejunum can be visualized, leaving most of the small intestine unexamined. The technique provides a diagnosis in a large percentage of patients with undiagnosed gastrointestinal bleeding (Figure 1) and enables us to treat it, especially in the case of vascular lesions.

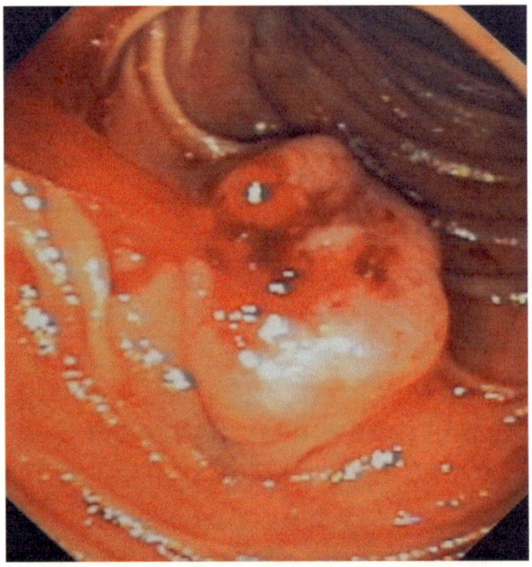

Fig. 1. Stromal tumor in the jejunum diagnosed using push enteroscopy.

Video capsule endoscopy. Visual capsule endoscopy is a noninvasive technique that has proven effective in the evaluation of patients with suspected bleeding of the small intestine. It enables us to visualize the whole small intestine. Several studies have proven the superiority of this technique over other conventional modalities, including barium x-ray. However, the real significance of specific findings and the false negatives caused by food and liquids, the lack of distension or propulsion, and the rapid passage through large segments are limitations that have yet to be resolved. The main disadvantage of the capsule is that it is an exclusively diagnostic technique, with limited capacity for identifying the lesion with accuracy and with no possibility of obtaining biopsies or carrying out therapeutic procedures (Figure 2).

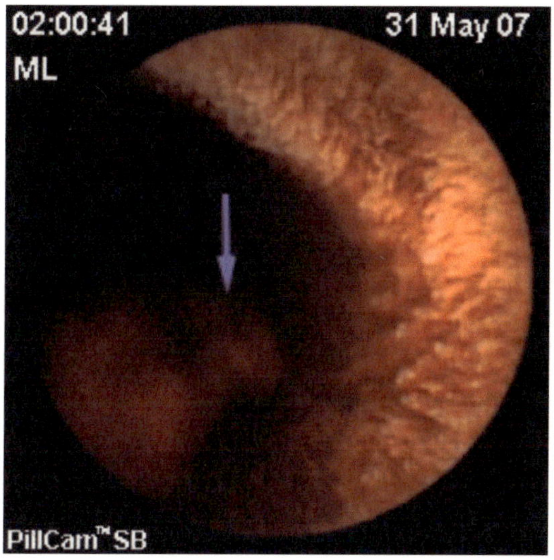

Fig. 2. Capsule endoscopy image of bleeding with a clot in the small intestine.

Balloon-assisted enteroscopy

a. *Double-balloon enteroscopy.* Double-balloon enteroscopy represents a huge advance. In theory, the whole small intestine can be examined, biopsies taken, and treatment administered, or, if this is not possible, the lesion can be marked. This technique makes it possible to reach more distal sections of the small intestine, although it rarely manages to reach the distal ileum; therefore, enteroscopy requires the combination of the antegrade and retrograde approaches for an examination of the whole intestine. Double-balloon enteroscopy is considered a safe and well-tolerated technique for the diagnosis and treatment of diseases of the small intestine.
b. *Single-balloon enteroscopy.* Single-balloon enteroscopy is the latest balloon-assisted endoscopic technique for the evaluation and management of small bowel disorders. It involves inserting a balloon catheter through the working channel of a colonoscope and moving the endoscope progressively along the small intestine by inflating and deflating the balloon. This technique has proven safe and effective, and in some cases (up to 25%) has made it possible to perform a complete enteroscopy.

Spiral enteroscopy. Spiral enteroscopy allows for advancement and withdrawal of the enteroscope through the small bowel by using clockwise and counterclockwise movements, respectively. The distal end of the overtube is positioned 25 cm from the tip of the enteroscope and locked into place. The system is then advanced to the ligament of Treitz with gentle rotation. The collar is subsequently unlocked, and the enteroscope is advanced past the ligament of Treitz. The overtube is then advanced using clockwise rotation until pleating of the small bowel no longer occurs over the enteroscope. The enteroscope is then unlocked and advanced to facilitate further advancement into the small bowel. In order to ease withdrawal of the enteroscope, the overtube is rotated in a counterclockwise direction. The insertion depth is 262±57 cm, and mean examination time is 33-35 minutes. This endoscopic modality also makes it possible to adopt a therapeutic approach, including biopsy, hemostasis, and polypectomy. Only minor complications (sore throat and minimal mucosal trauma) have been reported thus far and no perforations have been observed. Some studies have compared spiral enteroscopy with double-balloon enteroscopy and report that double-balloon enteroscopy has a better diagnostic yield.

Intraoperative enteroscopy. Intraoperative enteroscopy by insertion of an endoscope through 1 or more enterotomies has a high diagnostic yield, identifying lesions in 70-100% of patients. The technique is started once the surgeon has performed a laparotomy, in general to gain access to the small intestine. Once the small intestine is exposed, 2 or more enterotomies are made and the colonoscope is inserted with the surgeon's help. Intraoperative enteroscopy makes it possible to examine the whole small intestine, always with the assistance of a surgeon. It is limited by its high morbidity (intestinal wall hematoma, mesenteric hemorrhage, prolonged ileus, intestinal ischemia, and perforation); therefore, this procedure is reserved for patients with persistent bleeding and high transfusional requirements in whom diagnosis cannot be established by other means (Figure 3). A variation of the technique involves oral insertion of the enteroscope during surgery, which makes it possible to see 93% of the ileum and establish a diagnosis in almost 60% of cases. Its drawback is the considerable operative morbidity in a relatively high proportion of cases (serosal tear or ruptured mesenteric vein).

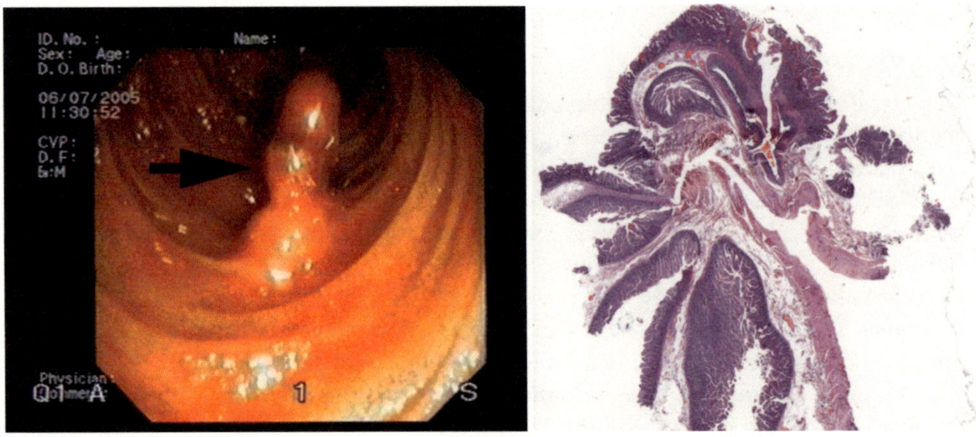

A. B.

Fig. 3. Jejunal aneurysm. A. Endoscopic image using intraoperative enteroscopy; B. Microscopic image showing caliber-persistent artery with mucosal rupture (x20)

5. Management of severe gastrointestinal bleeding

Severe bleeding in the small intestine is extremely problematic for a hospital. First, patient instability limits the diagnostic methods at our disposal. Second, not all hospitals have the diagnostic and therapeutic methods described here. Only tertiary hospitals can apply all the techniques described. Our objective should be to improve therapeutic options using the tools generally available in the hospital.

Consequently, when faced with a hemodynamically unstable patient who cannot be transferred, we must use all available diagnostic approaches, beginning with standard techniques (gastroscopy, colonoscopy, and helical CT) and moving on to other available methods such as intraoperative enteroscopy, which is indicated in acute intestinal bleeding of unknown origin, either when alternative techniques fail or when the patient's condition makes it impossible to apply them. Although this technique is very effective, in a small percentage of patients it may be impossible to find the bleeding source, especially when this is vascular and small. Nevertheless, it is still considered the reference technique, enabling accurate location of the lesion and minimally invasive surgery, with a lower number of recurrences.

It is very important to examine the whole small intestine, even once a lesion has been identified, as the presence of concomitant lesions could cause subsequent problems. Location of the lesion enables minimally invasive resection, with lower morbidity and mortality. In some cases with active bleeding, hemostasis can be restored using endoscopy. Once the patient is stable, the lesion can be resected.

Our approach to severe bleeding in the small intestine is to perform esophagogastroduodenoscopy and colonoscopy in order to rule out lesions in the corresponding areas. If the patient is sufficiently stable, capsule endoscopy can be performed and, depending on the location of the lesion, push enteroscopy or balloon-assisted enteroscopy can be used for therapy. If the lesion is not accessible for endoscopic treatment, a medical approach (embolization) or surgical approach should be adopted. If the patient presents massive bleeding or is hemodynamically unstable, CT angiography and/or arteriography are advised to locate and treat the cause of the bleeding. Intraoperative enteroscopy should be reserved for severe recurrent bleeding with high transfusion requirements, inaccessible lesions, or unavailability of balloon-assisted enteroscopy.

6. Summary

Total intraoperative enteroscopy is effective for the diagnosis of severe gastrointestinal bleeding of unknown origin. It enables more localized and efficacious surgery when other diagnostic techniques—arteriography, labeled red cell scintigraphy, and endoscopic capsule—cannot be performed. Furthermore, total intraoperative enteroscopy can be performed in selected cases at any hospital without the need for advanced technology.

7. References

Manning-Dimmitt LL, Dimmitt SG, Wilson GR. Diagnosis of gastrointestinal bleeding in adults. Am Fam Physician, 2005; 71: 1339-46.

Saperas E. Lower gastrointestinal bleeding: The great unknown. Gastroenterol Hepatol 2007; 30: 93-100.

Farrell JJ, Friedman LS. The management of lower gastrointestinal bleeding. Aliment Pharmacol Ther 2005; 21; 1281-98.

Brackman MR, Gushchin VV, Smith L, Demory M, Kirkpatrick JR, Stahl T. Acute lower gastroenteric bleeding retrospective analysis (the ALGEBRA study): An analysis of the triage, management and outcomes of patients with acute lower gastrointestinal bleeding. Am Surg 2003; 69: 145-9.

Mathus-Vliegen EM, Tytgat GN. Intraoperative endoscopy: Technique, indications, and results. Gastrointest Endosc, 1986; 32: 381-4.

Mihara Y, Kubota K, Nagata H, Takagi K, Hortie T, Oda N, et al. Total intraoperative endoscopy using acolonoscope for detecting the bleeding point. Hepatogastroenterology, 2004; 51: 1401-3.

Whelan RL, Buls JG, Goldberg SM, Rothenberger DA. Intraoperative endoscopy. University of Minnesota experience. Am Surg 1989; 55: 281-6.

Zaman A, Sheppard B, Katon RM. Total peroral intraoperative enteroscopy for obscure GI bleeding using a dedicated push enteroscope: diagnostic yield and patient outcome. Gastrointest Endosc 1999; 50: 506-10.

Douard R, Wind P, Panis Y, Marteau P, Bouhnik Y, Cellier C, et al. Intraoperative enteroscopy for diagnosis and management of unexplained gastrointestinal bleeding. Am J Surg 2000; 180: 181- 4.

Pérez Roldán F, González Carro P, Villafáñez García MC, Picazo Yeste J, Lucendo Villarín A. Urgent Intraoperative total enteroscopy with colonoscopy by means of a double enterotomy in a severe lower digestive tract haemorrhage. Cir Esp, 2009; 86: 252-3.

Akerman PA, Agrawai D, Cantero D, Pangtay J. Spiral enteroscopy with the new DSB overtube: a novel technique for deep peroral small-bowel intubation. Endoscopy, 2008; 40: 974-8.

Frieling T, Heise J, Sassenrath W, Hülsdonk A, Kreysel C. Prospective comparison between double-balloon enteroscopy and spiral enteroscopy. Endoscopy, 2010; 42: 885-8.

8

Transanal Endoscopic Operation - A New Proposal[1]

José Joaquim Ribeiro da Rocha[2] and Omar Féres[2]
[1]Division of Coloproctology of the Department of Surgery and Anatomy of Ribeirão Preto Faculty of Medicine – University of São Paulo (FMRP-USP),
[2]Division of Coloproctology of the Department of Surgery and Anatomy, Ribeirão Preto Faculty of Medicine – University of São Paulo (FMRP-USP),
Brazil

1. Introduction

In general, local excision (LE) is one of the many techniques available for rectal cancer treatment. When this technique is used on a selective group of tumors, the survival rates are similar to those of patients submitted to abdominal surgery resections. In patients with high surgical risk, the LE shows smaller morbidity and mortality, with also less anorectal, urinary and sexual function alterations [1-3].

The most commonly used techniques for LE include the colonoscopy with polypectomy loops, conventional transanal excision (CTE), transanal endoscopic microsurgery (TEM) and the posterior access surgery [4-7].

For local rectal cancer surgical treatment, the TEM has been used since 1983 with positive results, low recurrence rates and less post-operation complications compared to conventional procedures. The posterior access surgery presents a high complication rate and offers no advantage for villous tumor ressection that may be excised by transanal access techniques [8,9].

The pre-operative evaluation of candidates for a LE is of importance, since one must be certified that possible cure will be achieved by one of the proposed local surgical techniques. The rectal touch, rectoscopy, endorectal ultrasound and nuclear magnetic resonance are useful on the diagnosis and to determine the tumor stage on the pre- and post-operative times [10-14].Selection criteria represent a relevant factor on the LE success. However, specific criteria for these tumors selection are still not universally accepted [2,, 15-18]. Some parameters are indicated as requisites for determination of which tumors are theoretically adequate for transanal LE: smaller than 4 cm, mobile, restricted to only one quadrant, placed up to 10 cm of the anorectal line, well differentiated, with no lymphovascular or lymphonodal invasion, and endoscopic, tomographic and nuclear magnetic resonance evaluations that demonstrate that lesions are T1, T2 with no metastatic lesions [19].

The results of local treatment of rectal cancer are of difficult interpretation because the literature brings retrospective analysis of heterogeneous groups of patients, with different surgical indications and adjuvant therapies, while it lacks prospective homogeneous studies [1,20].

In our environment, the endoscopic transanal or surgical procedures for rectal tumors up to 15 cm of the anorectal line depend on the surgeon and/or endoscopist experience, on the equipment available and on the type of lesion. We use the CTE performed with anal retractors and basic surgical instruments for treatment of rectal lesions on the distal 1/3. The colonoscopy with polypectomy loops has allowed the resections of higher lesions, located on middle and superior rectum, on an appropriate manner.
The challenge comes when there is a benign, but of large volume and extension lesion, with or without carcinoma focuses, or on non invasive malignant neoplasms, located on middle or superior rectum, with no possibility for an endoscopic excision by colonoscopy and that can not be reached by CTE. In these circumstances, there is an indication for a transanal endoscopic surgery. In the absence of economic viability for the material acquisition, and surgical experience with complex methods like the TEM used by Buess [21,22] as also for the videoendoscopic transanal microsurgery (VETM) used by Swanstron [23] or the videoendoscopic transanal microsurgery without inflations [17,24-26] we have idealized, researched and executed a more simple technique, so called Transanal Endoscopic Operation (TEO).
In the present study, the main objective is to present the TEO as a method for local transanal excision of selected rectal lesions, and to present our clinical and surgical experience with this new method, comparing the results with those obtained with the well established endoscopic techniques available in the literature.

2. Casuistic and methods

We have designed a cylindrical rectoscope with 4 cm in diameter, with a 1 cm wide flap in one of the extremities, equidistantly perforated. In this flap, we attached a small (2 cm long) rectangular piece, of round contours, with a hole on the extremity and an aluminum screw on the base, used to fix it to the rectoscope flap (Fig. 1). This small piece is mobile and it is positioned in the way that its perforated extremity locates on the rectoscope lumen; in this position, the base screw is pressed and is used to hold the fiberlight cable, which will lighten the operative field (Fig. 2). The flap holes are used to fix the rectoscope with surgical thread to the anal border. In this way, with the rectoscope fixed to the anal border and the light correctly positioned, there is no need for an assistant surgeon for this task.

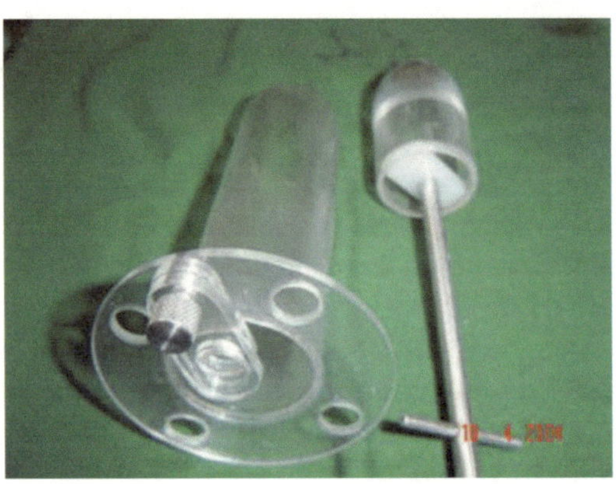

Fig. 1. Proctoscope presentation. Perforated flap and rectangular piece, of round contours, and the proctoscope guide

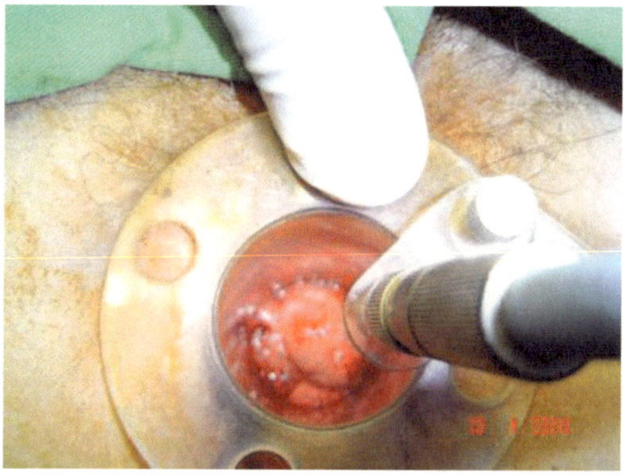

Fig. 2. Positioned proctoscope, together with the fixed fiberlight cable.

The equipment extremity which will be introduced has a beveled aspect and round borders (Fig 3). This format is very important for the essence of the procedure: since there is no inflations, this mechanical disposition allows the surgeon to position the rectoscope on the way that the longest part of this extremity holds the contra-lateral mucosa when the surgeon identifies the lesion, which will be now located on the center of the operative field.

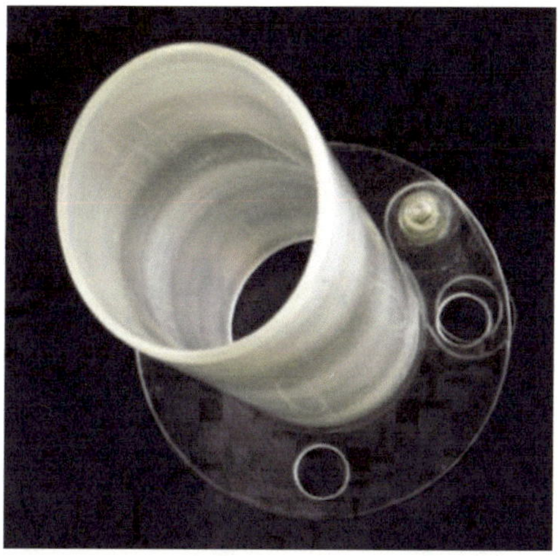

Fig. 3. Distal proctoscope end, showing the beveled aspect and round borders.

It is also part of the equipment a guide which will be positioned inside the rectoscope on the moment of its anal insertion (Fig. 1-4). It is composed of an aluminum cable with a round tip, being its caliber obviously smaller than the rectoscope´s one. On the tip of the guide there are two longitudinal ridges for air passage, avoiding the vacuum formation and the rectal mucosa aspiration during its removal from the rectoscope after its introduction.
Initially, only one 12 cm long rectoscope was built. After our experience with the equipment, another one, 20 cm long was built, once higher rectal lesions were also able to be removed with this method. Also, a smaller rectoscope (7 cm long) was built, which was ideal for excision of tumors located up to 5-6 cm from the anal border. Independently of the length, the rectoscopes contain all components described in this text.

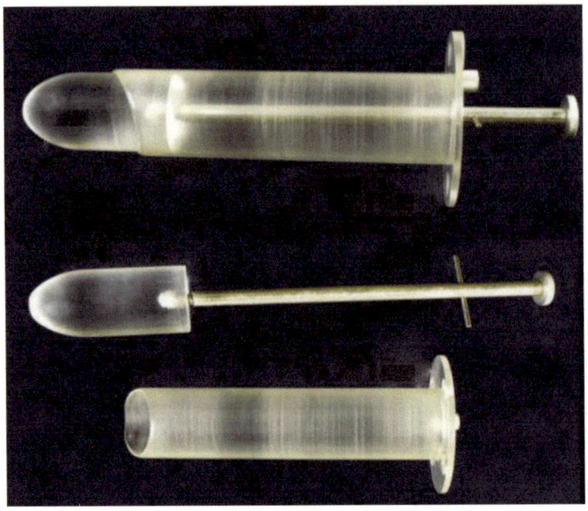

Fig. 4. Surgical proctoscopes (12 and 20 cm long) and respective guides.

Acrylic was chosen as the main equipment material, with small components in aluminum, for the following reasons: both these materials are easy to acquire, are of low costs, are easily manipulated by the staff who build the equipment in our facility and also because they are easy to be cleaned, disinfected and sterilized. More recently, a stainless steel rectoscope was built, more resistant and not transparent like the acrylic ones, with the advantage that the surgical field was lighter during its use (Fig. 5).

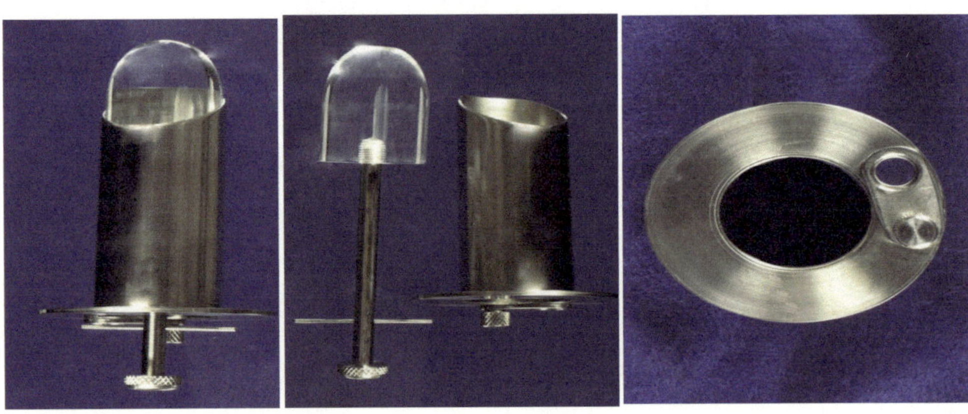

Fig. 5. Stainless steel rectoscopes

The accessories used for the TEO, together with the surgical rectoscope include a light source with a fiberlight cable (most of the times we used the light source from a videolaparoscopy equipment), an electrocautery with long pens and, when possible, also with thin tips to facilitate the lesion visualization, and forceps for holding and aspiration, used simultaneously. Other important components are: polypectomy loops, forceps for holding and presenting lesions (graspers), some of them from the videolaparoscopy equipment, long needle holders (conventional or from the videolaparoscopy equipment), long and thin aspiration tubes, syringes and suture threads.

2.1 Technical steps of the Transanal Endoscopic Operation (TEO)

Patients were prepared as for any other colorectal surgery: in the hospital, they receive clear liquid diet two days before the surgery, intestinal clearance with 10 % glycerin (retrograde preparation) or the oral use of osmotic laxatives (10 % manitol or sodium phosphate; anterograde preparation). Also, they are submitted to antibiotic therapy, beginning with i.v. metronidazole and ceftriaxona at the hospital and oral ciprofloxacin up to 7 days after surgery. All patients were regionally anaesthetized either by peridural (epidural) or spinal anesthesia, associated with i.v. sedation.

Operatory position was dependent on the rectal lesion location; posterior tumors were accessed through the litotomy position and anterior tumors were accessed though the "Jacknife" position.

After positioning the patient, antisepsis is done with topic PVP-I, surgical sheaths are placed, surgical tables and adequate surgical instruments are positioned, equipments such as light source, electrocautery and vacuum are checked and the anal dilation is carefully and manually performed, with topic lubrificant, until we get permeability for two fingers (usually the index and the middle fingers). The anus and anal canal are lubrified again with xylocaine 2% jelly before the rectoscope introduction. Two or three Allis forceps holding out the sphincters muscles might help the guide and the rectoscope penetration.

With gentle movements, the complete equipment, guide and body, is completely introduced up to the flap (Fig. 6). The guide is removed and the light source is connected to its place next to the flap. With an adequate view of the rectal lumen, the endoscope is positioned the way that the best exposition and presentation of the lesion are achieved (Fig. 7). In this situation, the equipment is fixed with cotton thread to the anal border.

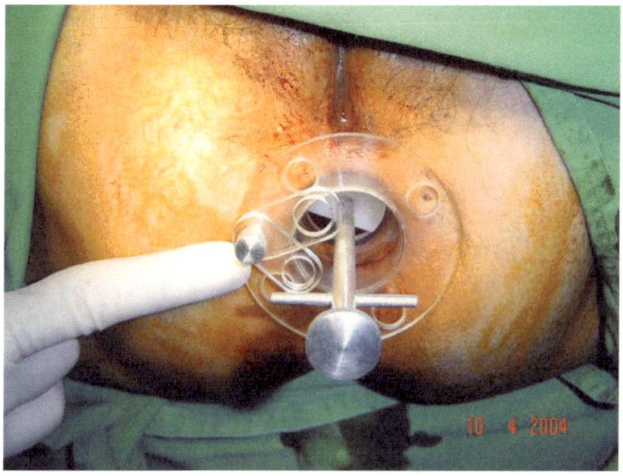

Fig. 6. Final aspect of the proctoscope and guide, after the correct introduction.

During the complete surgical procedure, saline irrigation and the electrocautery and vacuum are essential elements for the final result success. Observing the security limits (borders), adequate hemostasy and the resection deepness are also essential for a successful procedure.

After the lesion removal, which must be correctly oriented for the pathologist observation and diagnosis, a revision of the wound is performed. The last procedures of the TEO are saline and PVP-I irrigation, hemostasy and suture, before the rectoscope removal.

Vesical catheterization was performed only when there was post-operatory urinary retention and only for patient relief. Patients were kept in the hospital until they could accept normal oral diet and present signs of normal intestinal function, usually for 24 to 48 hours after surgery.

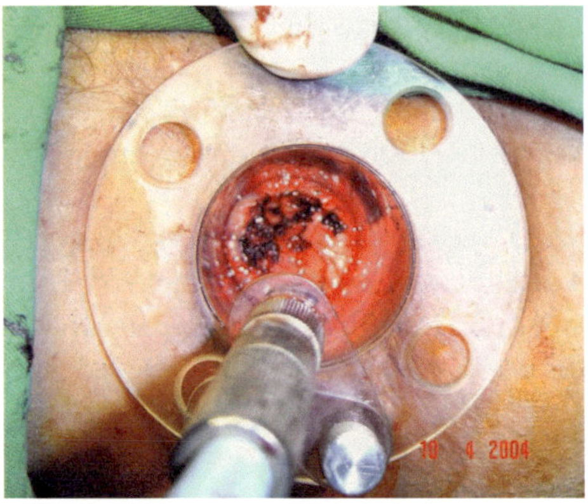

Fig. 7. Proctoscope surgically positioned and the correct presentation of the operatory field.

2.2 Evaluation of patients submitted to the Transanal Endoscopic Operation (TEO)

Eighty one patients submitted to the TEO, from August 2003 to February 2011 were included in the present study, being 36 patients from the Hospital São Paulo and 45 patients from the School of Medicine Hospital and Clinics, both in Ribeirão Preto City. The basic equipment and the surgeon was the same in all procedures.

A protocol with personal data, clinical history, previous history, physical, proctological and other exams, the indications for the TEO, performed procedures and clinical outcome was studied based on patients´ hospital records. In this protocol, data on surgical time, lesion anal distance, hospitalization time, intra-and post-operatory complications, follow up time, recurrence rates and posterior resections data were also studied.

Data obtained in this study was compared to data obtained by 39 different authors who used different techniques of TEO for transanal excision of rectal lesions. The metanalysis was used for the comparisons, a quantitative method whereby all data from all available studies of a determined subject are combined. Confidence intervals for proportions were obtained using the exact confidence interval for a proportion method [27]. Parameters analyzed by this method included the recurrence, complications and posterior resection rates. Recurrence rates were studied as total recurrence rate, adenoma recurrence rate and adenocarcinoma recurrence rate. For posterior resections, after the transanal excisions, the colorectal resection rates, so called rescue surgery, were quantified for all patients submitted to surgery and for patients with some kind of recurrence. Also, the rate for a new resection of local recurrence was evaluated.

Other data: lesion distance from the anorectal border, lesion size (on the widest diameter, in cm), operation time (in minutes), hospitalization time (in days), were described in scatter plot graphs, according to author and technique.

3. Results

3.1 Rectoscope idealized and built specifically for TEO

We consider successful the theoretical idea of building rectoscopes of 4 cm in diameter, with a fenestrated distal extremity and the proximal extremity with fixation and illumination supports. Because of the professional collaboration and support from our facility staff, associated with the financial support from the School of Medicine of Ribeirão Preto, there was no difficulty in projecting and building the ideal equipment for the TEO. In the time frame of 3 months, the ideal equipment was built and ready to use.

3.2 The Transanal Endoscopic Operation (TEO)

Eighty three patients were selected to be submitted to the TEO, with the described proctoscope. In two of these patients the TEO was not performed: one because of anal stenosis and the other because the lesion was more than 15 cm from the anal border, in an angulated area. The TEO, following the technical steps described previously, was successfully performed on the other 81 patients.

3.3 Evaluation of the patients submitted to the TEO

The table 1 shows the literature review of techniques used for local excision of rectal lesions, used for comparisons with the proposed TEO. Four studies were excluded from this analysis because there were not enough data for a comparative analysis. In this way, 35 different studies, being 26 of TEM, 4 of two or more techniques, 3 of VETM and 2 of CTE were compared. Because not all authors have cited all parameters compared in the present study, the scatter plots that illustrate the comparisons do not always present 35 points.

Number	Used techniques	Author(s)/year
1	CTE	Budhoo & Hancok, 2000
2	CTE	Aguilar, 2000
3	CTE-TEM- posterior access	Balani, 2000
4	CTE- posterior access	Graham, 1999
5	CTE-TEM	Morschell, 1998
6	TEM	Mentges, 1996
7	TEM	Mentges, 1996
8	TEM	Mentges, 1997
9	CTE-TEM	Stipa, 2005
10	TEM	Salm, 1994
11	TEM	Said, 1992
12	TEM	Steele, 1996
13	TEM	Lezoche, 1996

Number	Used techniques	Author(s)/year
14	TEM	Winde, 1998
15	TEM	Heintz, 1998
16	TEM	Doornebosch, 1998
17	TEM	Yamasaki, 1999
18	TEM	Ikeda, 2000
19	TEM	Lev-Chelouche, 2000
20	TEM	Arribas del Amo, 2000
21	TEM	Demartines, 2000
22	TEM	Ziprin, 2002
23	TEM	Farmer, 2002
24	TEM	Lloyd, 2002
25	TEM	Marks, 2003
26	TEM	Cocilovo, 2003
27	TEM	Lee, 2003
28	TEM	Neary, 2003
29	TEM	Kattri, 2004
30	TEM	Stipa, 2004
31	TEM	Meng, 2004
32	TEM	Palma, 2004
33	TEM	Endreseth, 2005
34	TEM	Duek, 2005
35	TEM	Rokke, 2005
36	VETM I	Swanstrom, 1997
37	VETM II	Nakagoe, 2003
38	VETM II	Araki, 2003
39	EMR	Hurlstone, 2005
40	TEO	Rocha, 2004

CTE: Conventional transanal excision
TEM: Transanal endoscopic microsurgery
VETM: Video endoscopic transanal microsurgery
EMR: Endoscopic mucosal ressection
TEO: Transanal endoscopic operation

Table 1. Relation between most commonly used techniques and respective authors.

3.4 Recurrence rates evaluation (average proportions)

Adenoma recurrence rates

From 11 references compared, only one is out of the confidence interval for the TEO, showing a smaller recurrence rate for adenomas (Graph I).

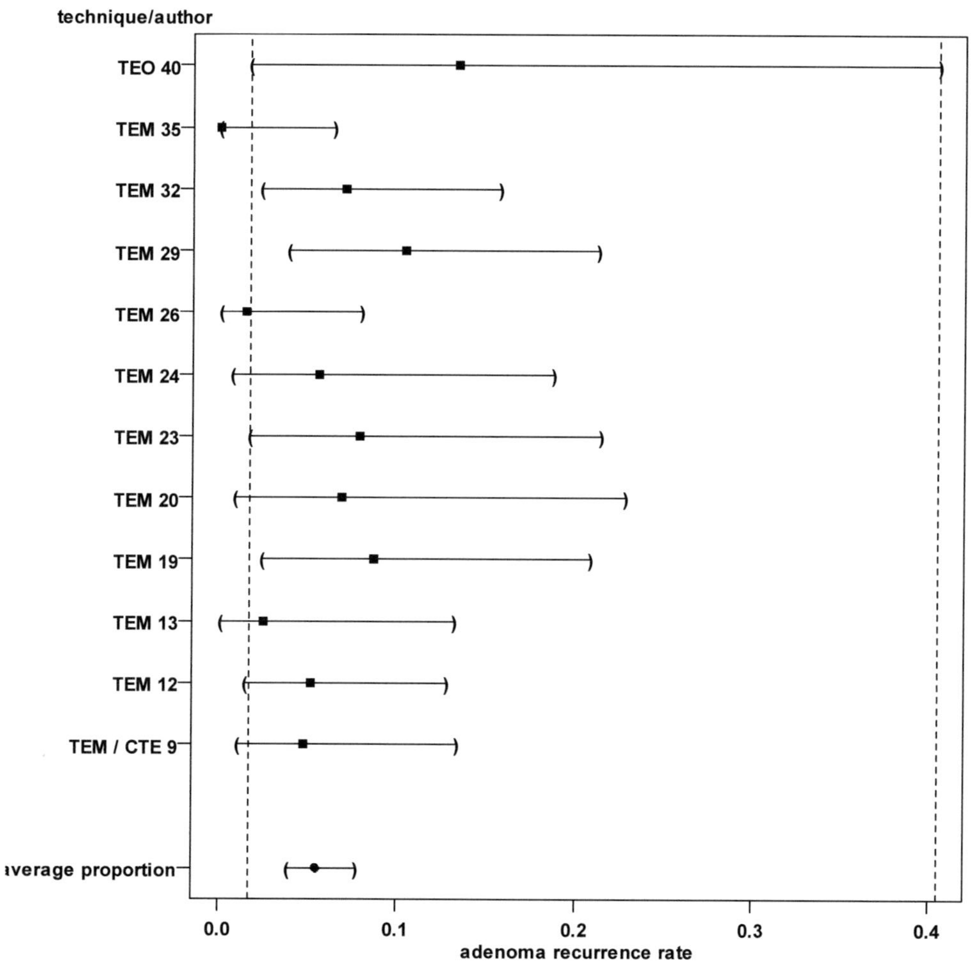

Graph 1. Adenoma recurrence rates.

Adenocarcinoma recurrence rates

The TEO showed two adenocarcinoma recurrence and among 17 compared references, 6 present rates higher that the maximum confidence interval accepted (Graph II).

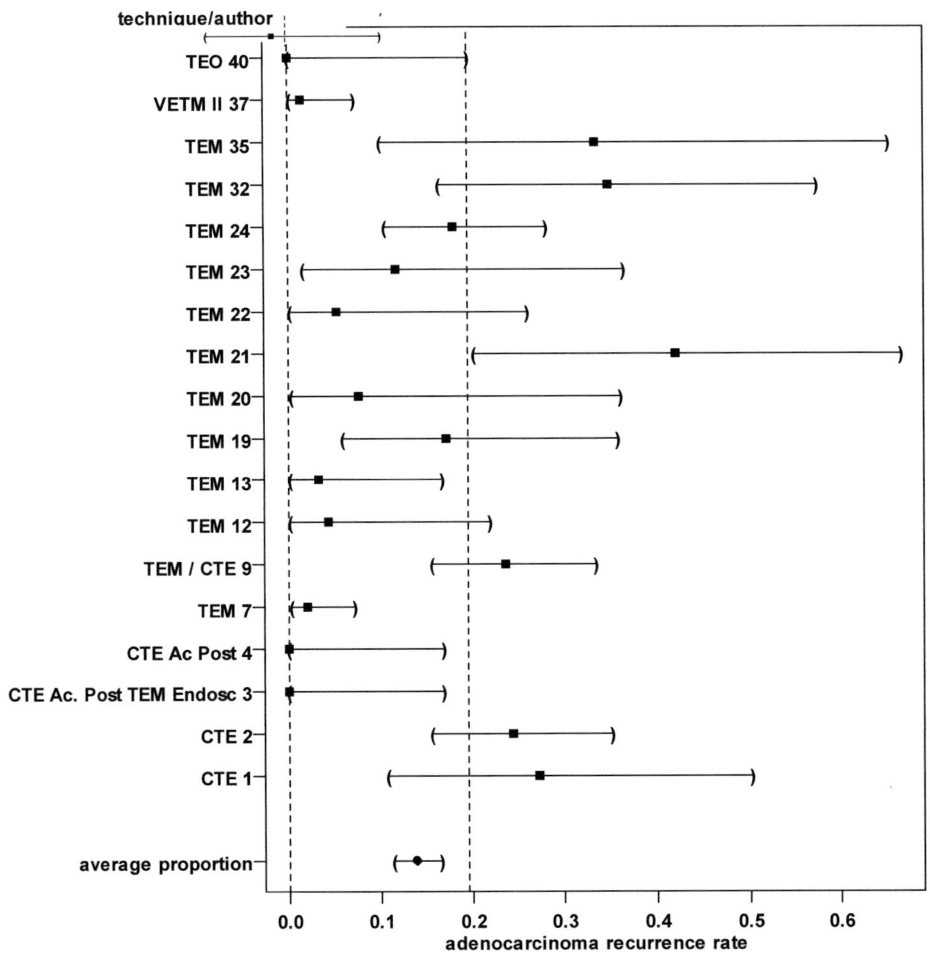

Graph 2. Adenocarcinoma recurrence rates

Total recurrence rates

Twenty-five references were selected for this comparison with TEO. Seven of them presented smaller total recurrence rates, out of the TEO confidence interval while 3 presented higher rates. Most of them (15) are on the confidence intervals expected for the TEO (Graph III).

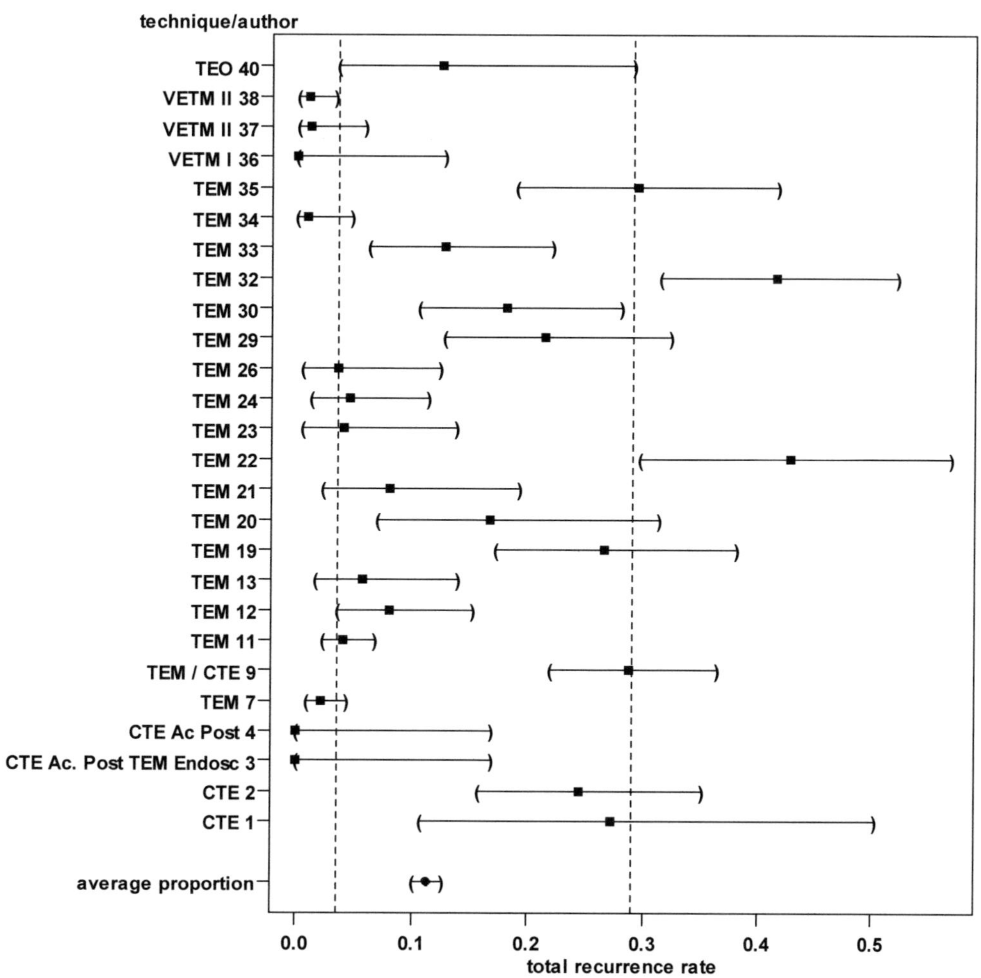

Graph 3. Total recurrence rates.

3.5 Complication rates evaluation (average proportions)

Only four in 28 references used for the analysis were out of the TEO confidence interval. Twenty-four of them present similar average proportions, and confidence intervals of the TEO (Graph IV).

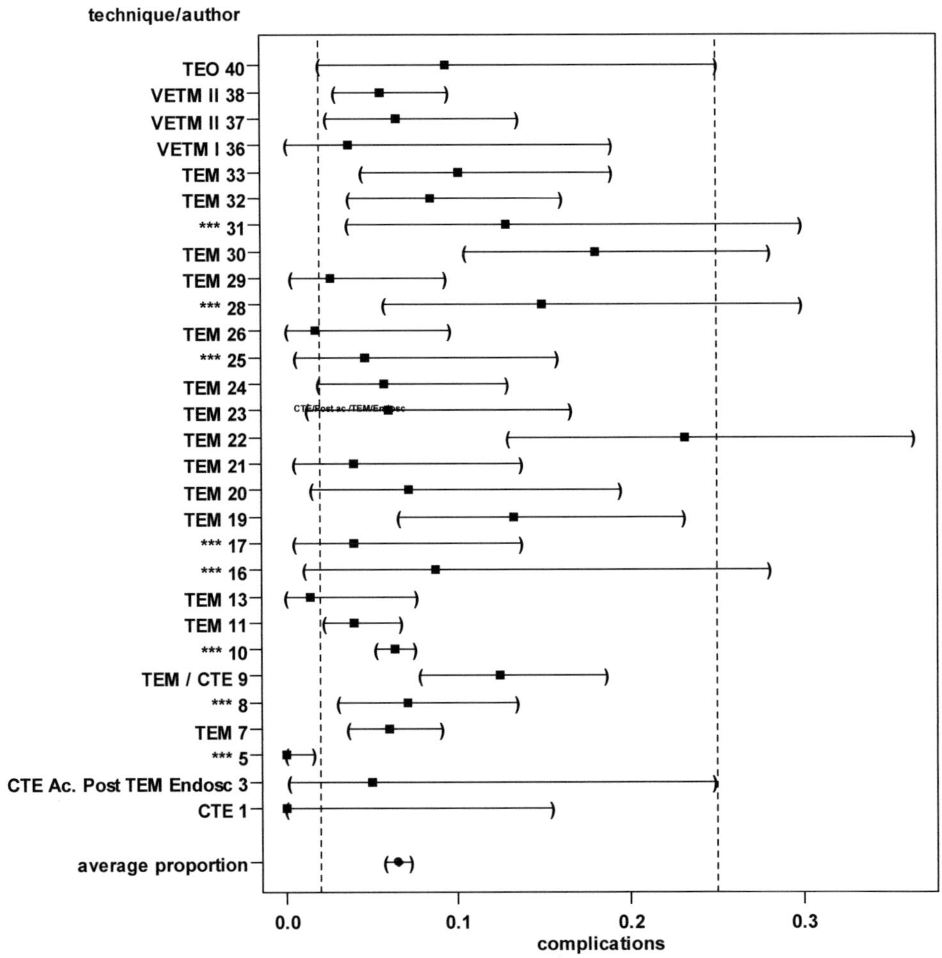

Graph 4. Complication rates.

3.6 Posterior colorectal resections rate evaluation (average proportions)

Colorectal resection rates in all patients

With the exception of one reference which is over the maximum confidence interval for the TEO, the other 13 evaluated show similar average proportions in the TEO confidence intervals. Average proportion of all references is 0.06 (Graph V).

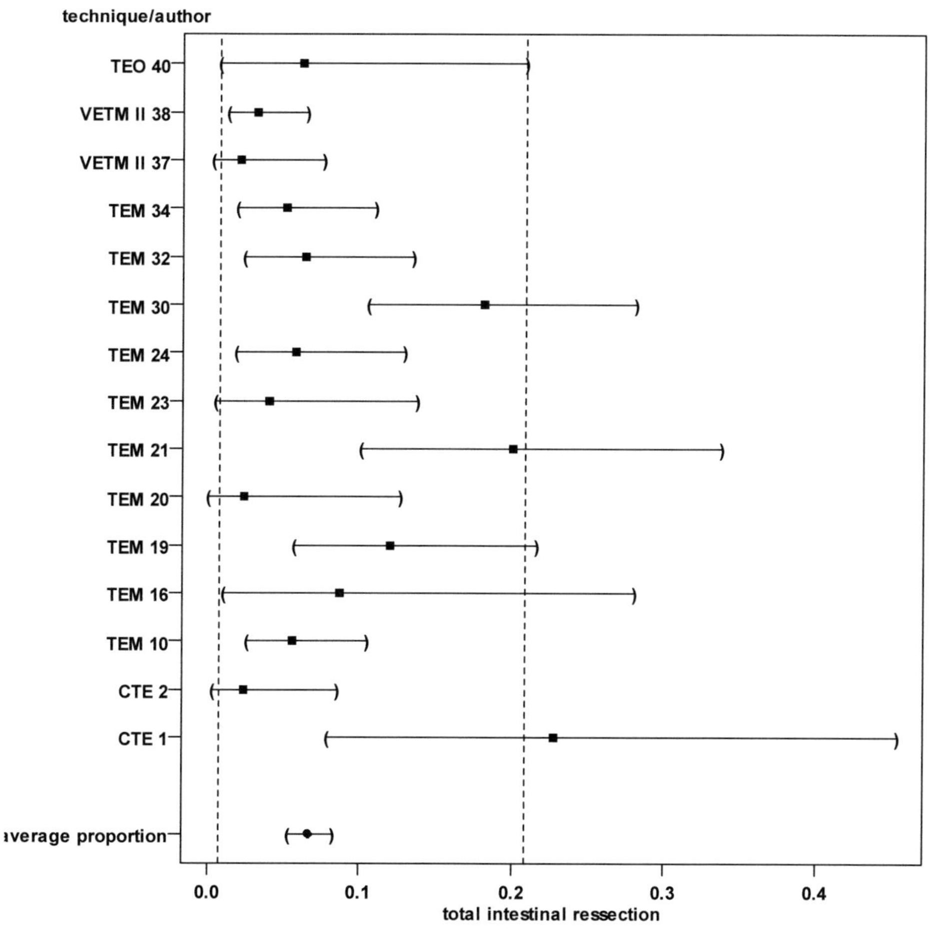

Graph 5. Colorectal resection rates in all patients.

Recurrence colorectal resections rates

In this analysis, the average proportion of all cases is of 0.5. From the 12 evaluated references, only one showed a smaller rate than the minimum confidence interval for the TEO and other 3 showed average proportions higher than the maximum confidence interval (Graph VI).

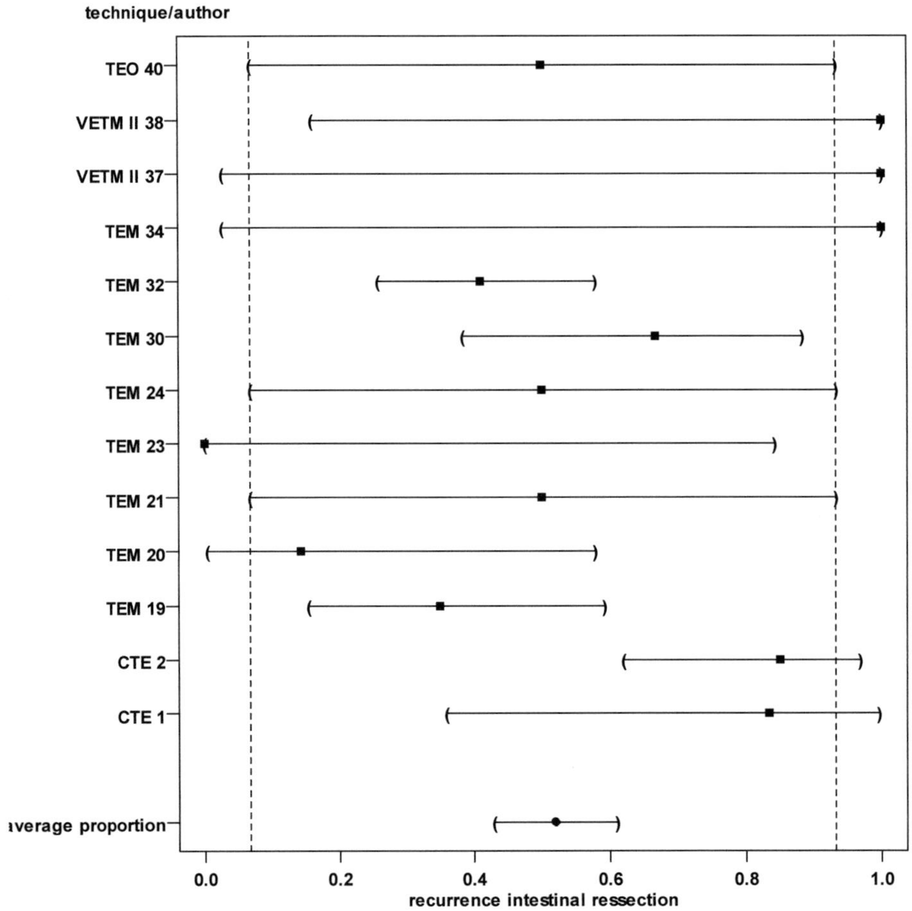

Graph 6. Recurrence colorectal resections rates.

New resection of local recurrence rates

Only six references were available for this comparison. Half of them showed average proportions smaller than the TEO and only one showed a high value, larger than the maximum confidence interval of the TEO (Graph VII).

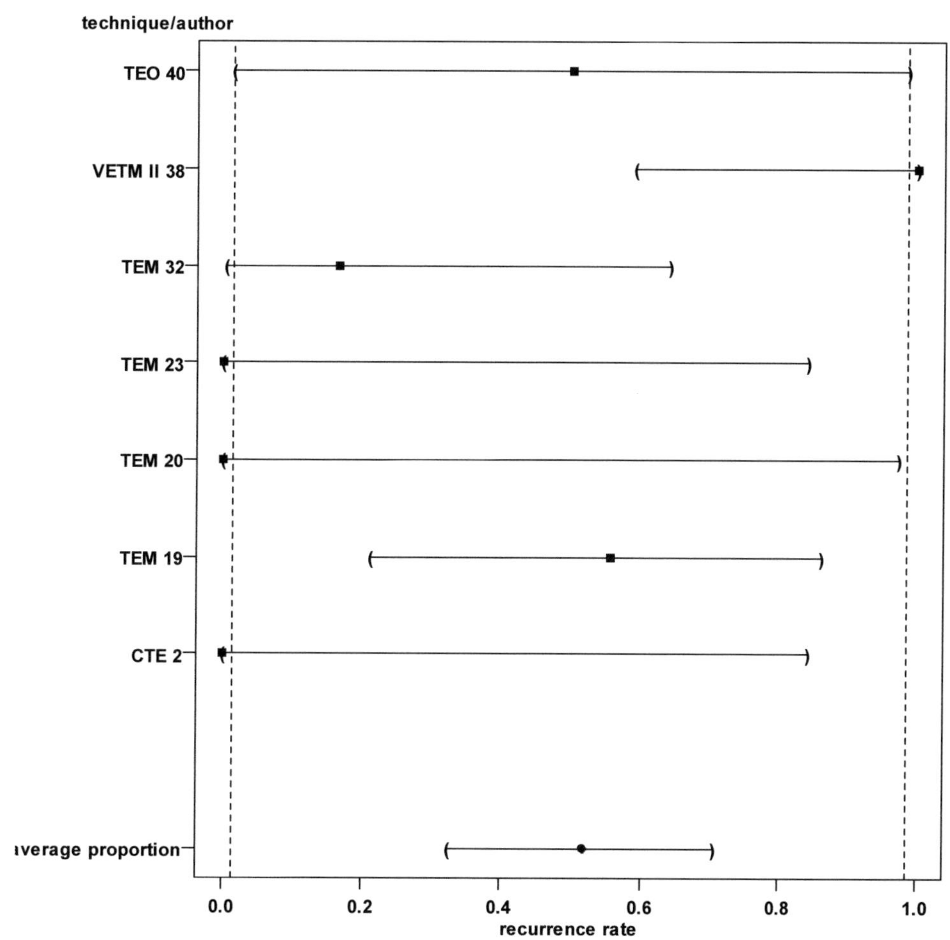

Graph 7. New resection of local recurrence rates.

3.7 Average distance from the anal border evaluation

This data is presented on graph VIII. Seven references described these values, being the values between 12 and 5cm.The TEO values averaged 7.3cm.

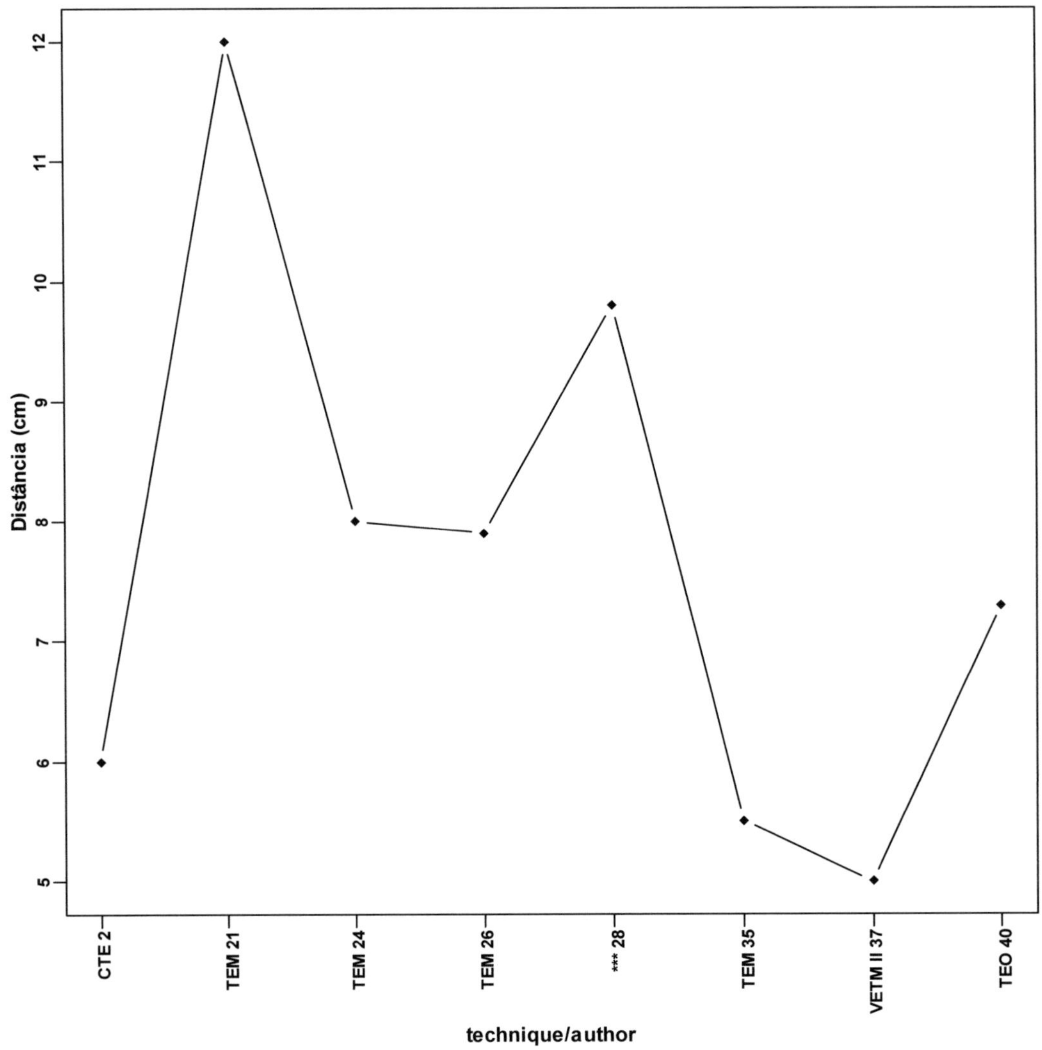

Graph 8. Average distance from the anal border evaluation.

3.8 Average lesion size evaluation (wider diameter)

The average diameter of the excised lesions with TEO was 3.6 cm. Maximum size was 4.9 cm and minimum size was 2.0 cm in the literature compared (Graph IX).

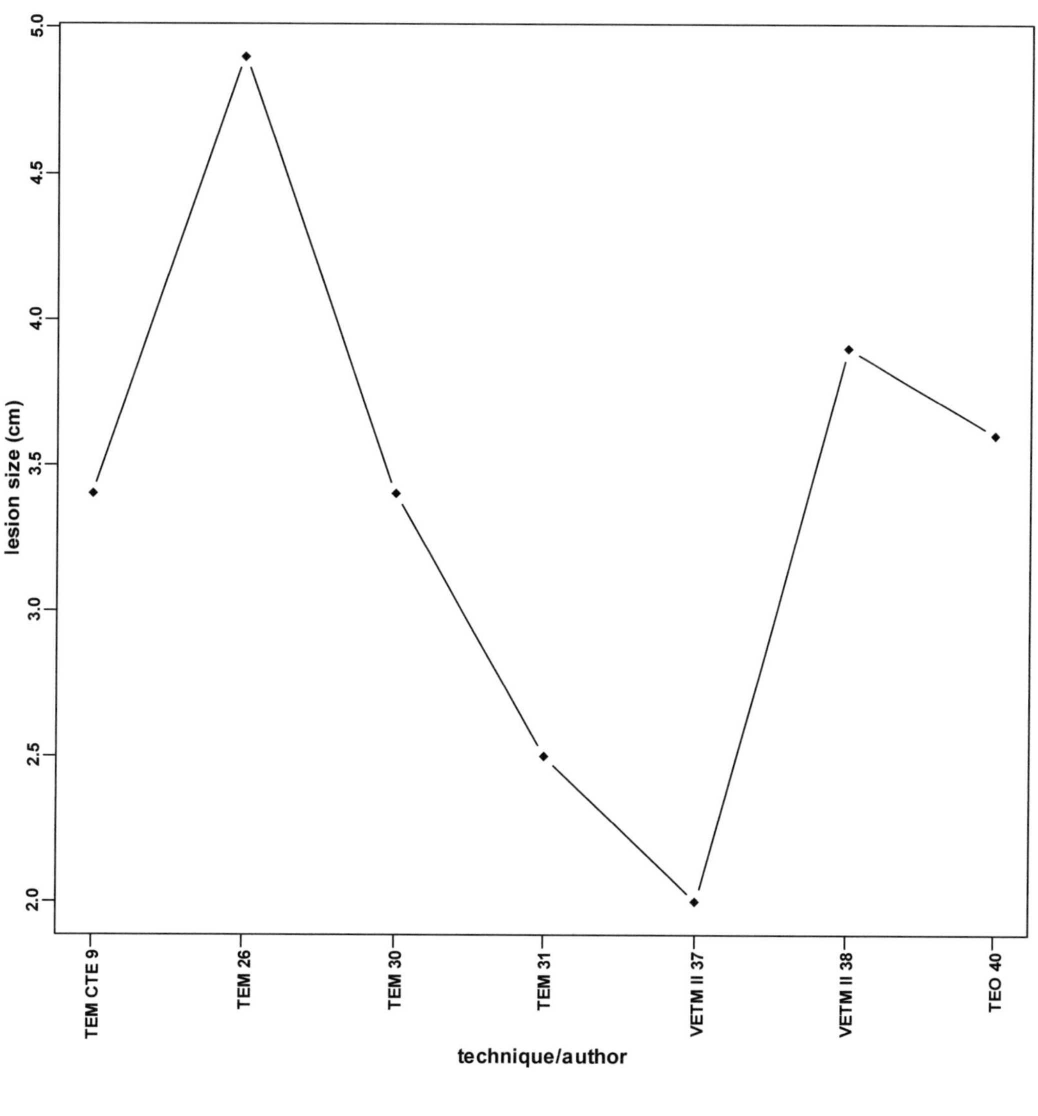

Graph 9. Average lesion size evaluation (wider diameter).

3.9 Surgical time evaluation

Eleven references were compared and the maximum average described was 175 minutes while the smaller average described was 53 minutes. The TEO average time was 56 minutes (Graph X).

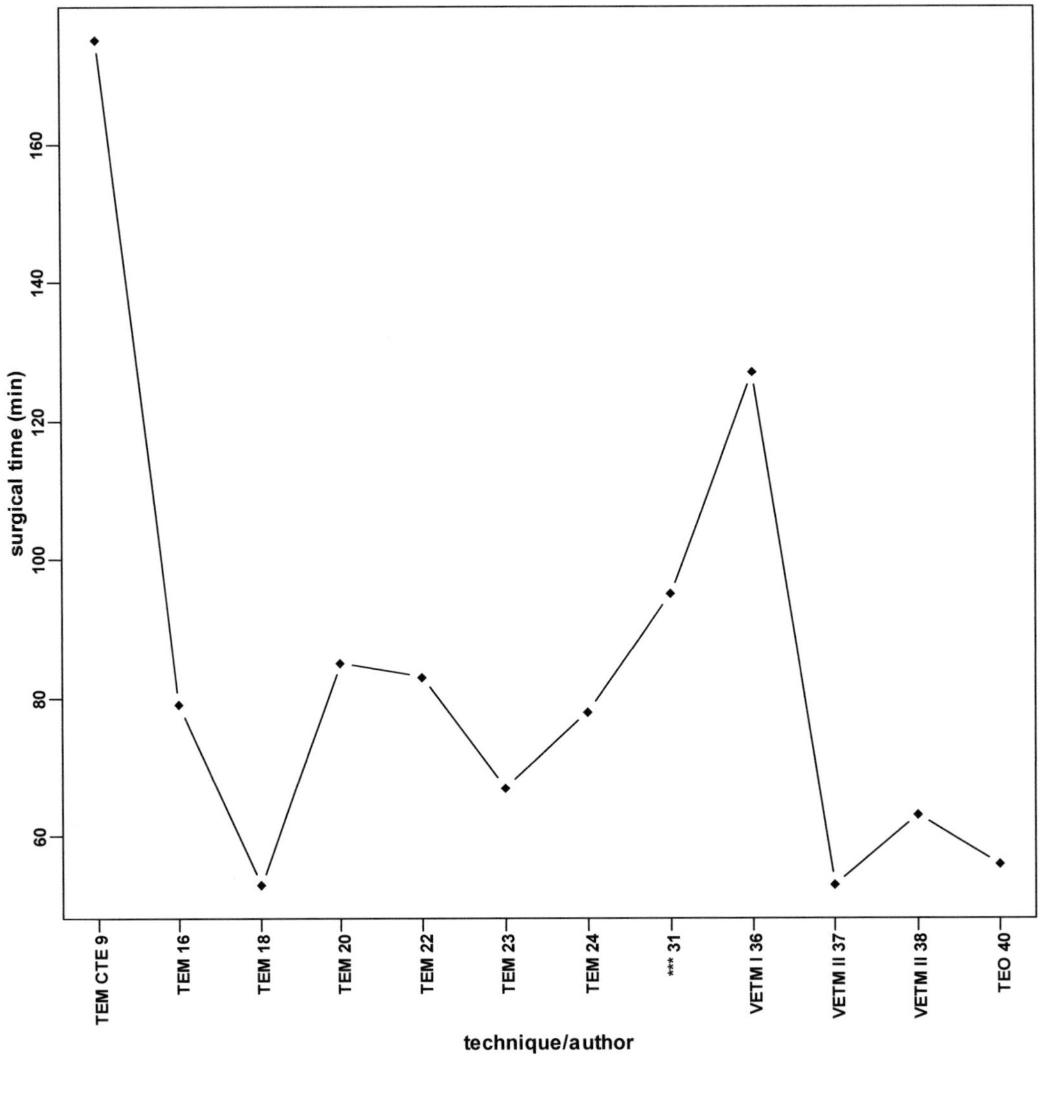

Graph 10. Surgical time evaluation.

3.10 Average hospitalization time

The smaller average presented in seven references was the TEO data of 2.4 days. The higher value was 5.8 days on average (Graph XI).

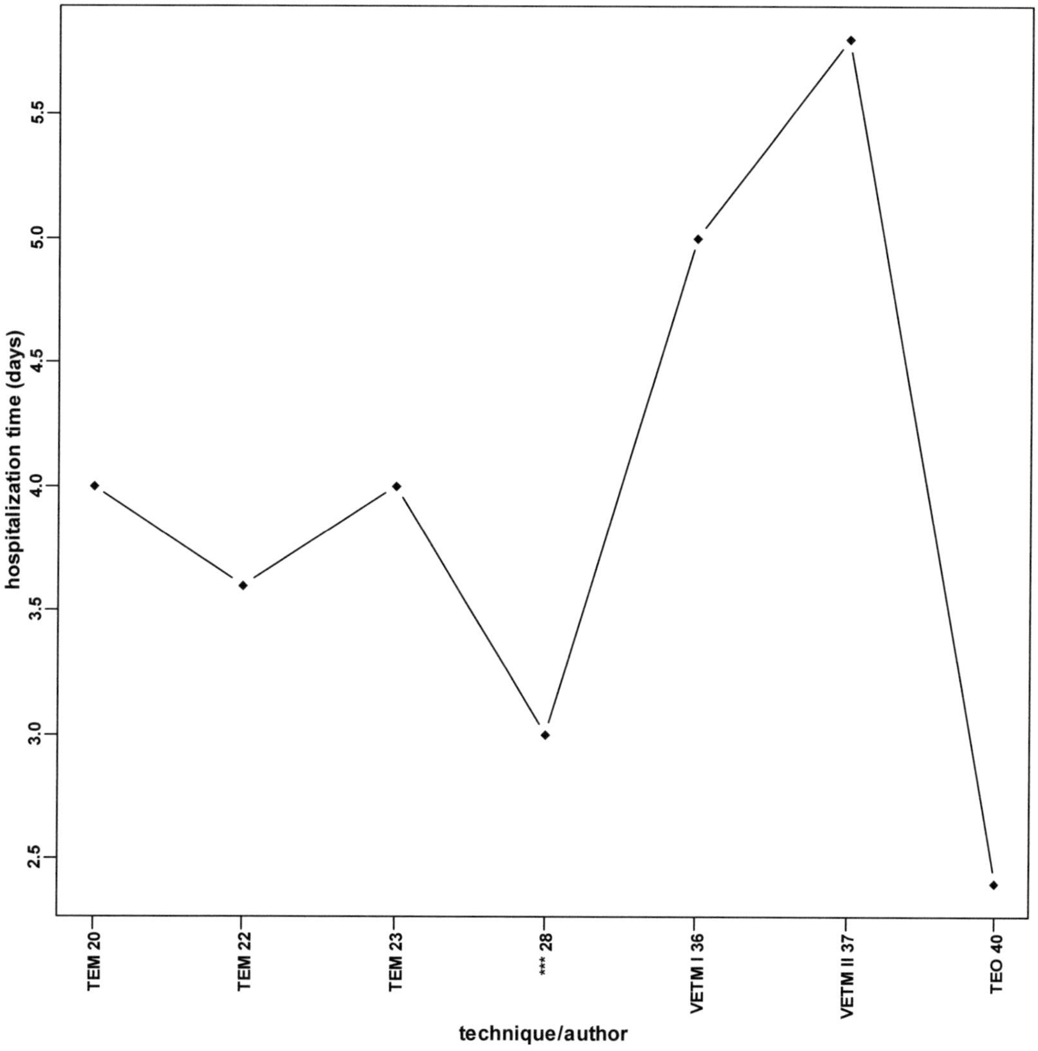

Graph 11. Average hospitalization time.

3.11 Follow up average time

The longest follow up period was 10 years. From the 26 references, 11 presented follow up times of 3 years or less our average varied from 2 months to 8 years (Graph XII).

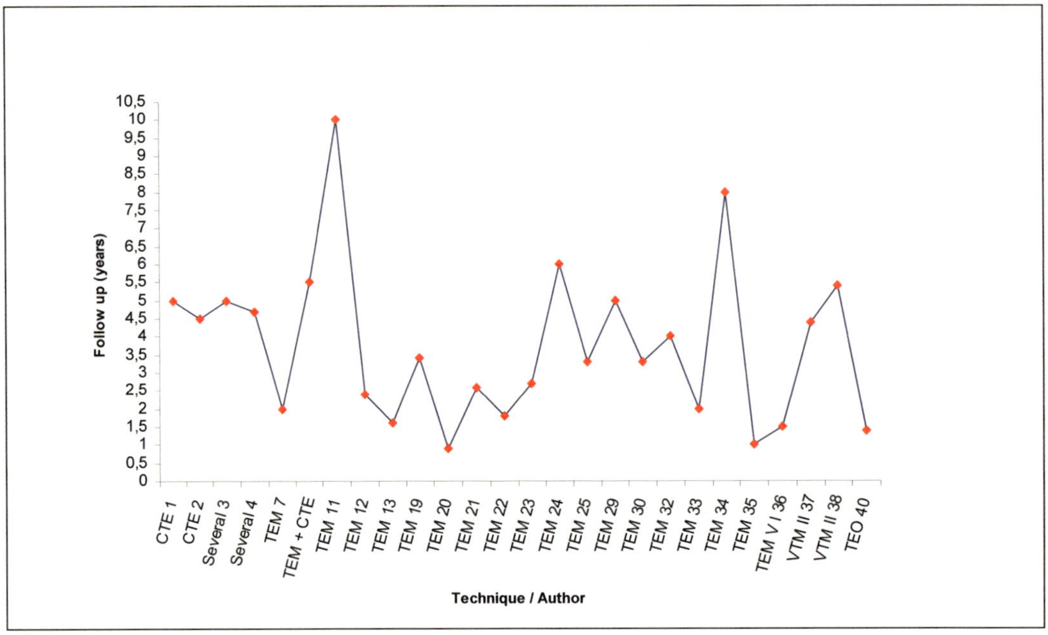

Graph 12. Follow up average time.

4. Discussion

Local excision of rectal tumors is a well established procedure as a surgical method. It is a less invasive procedure that, according to its indication criteria, brings benefits in terms of rectal and canal anal functional preservation, morbid-mortality and costs [1,2].

Literature estimates reveal that 40 to 50 % of the primary rectal cancer will be presented without lymphonodal commitment (T1, T2, T3 - No) as soon as diagnosed [27,28] and that 15% of the patients considered cured show tumors limited to the rectal wall (T1 - T3 - No) [29]. Every year, more than 7000 patients with rectal cancer are potentially cured by local excision as the only therapeutic method [30].

Proctological exam (clinical and rectoscopy), the USER and MRI are important on the selection of patients to be submitted to transanal excision [3,7,13,14].

Classic and reasonable indications for rectal tumors local resection include T1, T2 mobile tumors, with adequate histological aspects (well or moderately differentiated, with no angiolymphatic invasion) [16-18].

Some references comparing transanal excision and radical resections demonstrated that low risk T1 lesions present similar survival and recurrence rates, with local excision, showing smaller hospitalization and surgical time, less analgesia and blood loss and less early and late morbidities. Data on T2 lesions are controversial [31-34]. Benign lesions are also included, especially the villous or tubulo-villous adenomas which resection was not possible by means of colonoscopy or conventional transanal excision.

We believe that, in diagnosing a rectal neoplasm lesion within or close to the transanal resection criteria, the complete resection is the logical conduct, which will allow a better histopathological evaluation than the regular biopsy.

It is not the tumor size or form but how deep it invades the wall and its malignant histological characteristics that will guide the final decision of a local excision. On the possibility of a complete lesion removal by local excision, this should be the first option. The decision for a large surgery depends on a good relation between the surgeon and the pathologist [35].

For the inferior or middle third rectal mobile tumors, technically accessible by the local excision, we suggest the excision to be done as "total biopsy", considering this method as the best one for their treatment. The "total biopsy" may constitute the definitive treatment for patients carefully selected.

On the presence of factors suggestive of bad prognosis, such as a deep lesion throughout the intestinal wall, incomplete surgical excision, presence of undifferentiated cells, venous or lymphatic invasion, and mucinous tumors, more aggressive and radical surgeries are indicated [36]. The final therapeutic decision must not be done before the complete examination of the tissue [9].

The advantage of having a tissue sample for the histopathological exam has been a stimulus for a complete local excision in selected patients. If we are sure that the cancer is not invasive, all efforts must be done in order to preserve the sphincter function.

In this way, the local excision of the complete lesion is the logical procedure, much better than just the biopsy because it allows: 1- the whole sample histopathological evaluation, 2- a chance for cure with a minimal invasive procedure, 3- on the necessity of a radical surgery, there was no prejudice for the patient, 4- the histopathological evaluation of this "total biopsy" will guide the further therapeutic proposal.

There are several procedures for local excision of rectal tumors. The conventional transanal excision (CTE), performed with anal retractors, is acceptable for lesions on the distal third of the rectum up to 4 cm in diameter. Posterior access, by means of transsacral or transsphincteric excisions do not offer advantages compared to the transanal techniques and have been less commonly used in the last decades [9].

Minimally invasive methods for rectal tumor resection with the use of rectoscopes are well accepted, widely used and improved in terms of technique in the last two decades. The transanal endoscopic microsurgery (TEM) idealized and preconized by Buess [37,38], is used in different countries: Germany, Italy, United Kingdom, Japan, Israel, Spain, Swiss, Australia, China, USA and others. Since its introduction into the clinical practice, some innovations were added to the technique, in order to improve the final performance of the procedure. Among the TEM innovations are some different types (modalities) of the endoscopic access, mainly aimed in order to reduce the equipment costs.

The first modification of the original TEM was proposed by Swanstron [23] where the authors propose the use of the videolaparoscopy equipment; this technique is known as video-endoscopic Transanal Microsurgery (VETM). In sequence, Japanese surgeons have modified the VETM performing it without gas inflation. These two main modifications of the original technique reduced the equipment price in approximately US$ 50000.00 [24-26, 39].

Despite that the literature on the local excision of rectal tumors indicates high survival rates and good results about the local control of the disease, selection criteria for patient are restrict. Only about 3 to 8% of invasive rectal tumors are qualified for this kind of treatment, based on those criteria [36,40].

From all available techniques for local excision of rectal lesions, the endoscopic procedures (TEM and others) are the most internationally used. Nevertheless, these techniques demand experience and, in consequence, must be performed in reference centers where a larger number of patients are available, facing that the surgeon training is mandatory and the small frequency of the indications is a reality [41-44]. Because of the necessity of having specific instruments and also the particular technical aspects, this method demands good training for the obtention of satisfactory results [45-47]. It was described that in 11 tumors located up to 4 cm of the anorectal line, a surgical conversion was necessary because of technical difficulties [48]. Due to two important disadvantages: first the high costs, taking into account the limitation of the equipment use and second, technical difficulties to perform the technique with ability and efficiency, the procedure has not achieved wide acceptance and popularity [23,49].

In Brazil, very few surgeons use the TEM technique proposed by Buess.

Due to the explained circumstances and facing the reality of a growing consecutive series of the distal third rectal neoplasm, with most of them committing old patients, with relevant comorbidities and high surgical and anesthetic risks, we started thinking of a less invasive alternative procedure than the radical abdominal resections, which would be more efficient than the conventional transanal excision and less complicated than the posterior accesses.

In this way, we proposed the TEO: we idealized and built a surgical proctoscope of low costs, associated to conventional surgical instruments, a fiberlight source, polipectomy loops and videolaparoscopic forceps, without the necessity of inflation or video cameras. The equipment built in our precision tool facility (Oficina de Precisão da Faculdade de Medicina de Ribeirão Preto - Hospital das Clinicas) showed very good results. From the 83 proposed surgeries, in only two it was not possible to conclude the procedure, one due to a rectal stenosis and the other due to the distance of the lesion from the anal border (15 cm), with an accentuated rectal-sigmoidal angle.

On the opposite way from the other transanal endoscopic techniques, mainly the TEM, which are inefficient for the excision of the inferior third rectal tumors because it is not possible to keep the equipment on the rectal lumen under inflation [50], on the TEO, with the 7 cm rectoscope, these lesions were easily excised.

With the increasing surgeon experience, it was possible to modify the rectoscope making it easier to handle and the surgical steps efficient and fast. These modifications included the use of the stainless steel as the main component, the 0.5 cm enlargement in the rectoscope diameter and the reduction of the electrocautery and vacuum tubes tips. This idealized proctoscope showed to be a very useful tool, with low cost, easy to handle and that allowed the obtaining of reliable results, similar to those already described for other transanal endoscopic techniques.

On the casuistic of the present study, six cases previously submitted to one or two endoscopic excision by means of colonoscopy (two superficial adenocarcinoma three villous-adenomas) were successfully submitted to the TEO. Another patient with villous-adenoma and high grade dysplasia, previously submitted to an CTE and presenting a recurrent lesion was also successfully submitted to the TEO. Eight patients were submitted to the TEO twice, or for the complete excision of the tumor or to the excision of residual or recurrent lesion suspect tissue.

The comparative results presented by the several local excision techniques are difficult to interpret since most of literature descriptions are based on retrospective analysis and on heterogeneous groups. Also, there is no randomized prospective studies and there is a lot of variation concerning the adjuvant therapy indication [1,2,16,17,20].

Another relevant aspect for literature data comparison is the biological characterization of the tumor, i.e., interaction tumor-host, which might be inferred by the morphology, histology, size, localization and invasive stage. This is essential for the therapeutic results comparison in patients with similar disease stages [51].

The lack of homogeneity in the literature is due to the difficulty in having a large number of patients for the study and also due to the necessity of classifying them according to the tumor stage (Tis, T1, T2, T3). Some authors use radiotherapy and others don't; while some authors exclude from the recurrence statistics those patients operated by local excision and, after diagnosing that the resection borders still had tumor, were right after submitted to a radical resection.

Despite recognizing the difficulties to find reports with the necessary severity for closer comparisons with the reality, 35 reviews were compared aiming the objectives of the present study.

We consider our recurrence rate very favorable since, to the moment only two recurrence were observed for the curative adenocarcinomas excised with TEO. For the adenomas, the average observed in our study is compatible with the literature revised, except one (Graphs I and II). If we group both rates on the total recurrence rate, the results are also similar to the literature (Graph III). These observations indicate that we should keep the surgery indication criteria, and continue to improve the technique and to observe the patients for a longer period of time.

The post-operatory complications were observed in total since the literature available does not discriminate in mild or severe complications. Our complications rate is acceptable (Graph IV) and compatible with most of the literature revised. In two cases there was a severe complication (pneumoretroperitoneum) on the 5th and 3rd post-operatory day. The first patient was operated on for a distal rectum opening on a patient with invasive, advanced and obstructed neoplasm and in this particular case a re-intervention was necessary, with a loop sigmoidostomy. The other case was treated conservatively and had good response There was one pneumoperitoneum after a second TEO for a recurrent villous adenoma, when the peritoneal fold was opened, treated clinically, the patient had a good response. Other complications such as pain, evacuation bleeding, urinary difficulties, were treated clinically.

The average proportions of the intestinal resections after local excisions are small and equivalent to the literature (Graph V). The observations of the intestinal resections after neoplasm lesions recurrence were ten times larger but also comparable to the literature (Graph VI).

In our study, two patients were re-operated (intestinal resections) after the TEO: one with a resting villous-adenoma 15 cm above the anorectal border, not reached with the surgical rectoscope, and the other one with an adenocarcinoma on the rectal mid third, with angiolymphatic invasion and compromised border, who was submitted to a total proctocolectomy. Nevertheless, the folowing histopathological exam did not show the presence of neoplasm on the tissue.

The results of a second local excision due to a residual lesion or recurrence demonstrated that performing another local excision or an intestinal resection it is still controversial since half of the revised literature has shown average proportions inferior to the TEO (Graph VII).

In the present study we performed four TEO re-operations being the indication based on the fibrosis and suspect granulation on the lesion border but in both cases, the histopathological analysis did not show resting neoplasm.

For some variables of interest, the correlation between or results and the literature were analyzed (Graphs VII to XII). These variables were the distance of the lesion from the anal border, lesion size represented by its maximum diameter, operation time ant hospitalization time.

The evaluation of the anal border distance of the lesions allows us to infer that the local excision is safely performed on the mid and inferior thirds of the rectum. In the literature, there are reports of TEM excisions of 15 to 18 cm lesions. In the present study we reached tumors up to 12 cm. Only one case of a lesion located 15 cm from the anal border was not reached due to a rectal-sigmoidal angulation.

The lesion size analysis, expressed in cm in its maximum diameter, showed very good results since, in our study, lesions up to 7 cm were excised. Other authors refer the excision of 8-9 cm lesions but this situation is related to those giant villous-adenomas, in which the endoscopic resections might be done in more than one surgical time.

The analysis of Graph X indicates that TEO shows a very short operative time, which is probably due to the fact that the equipment is simple and easy to use and that the procedure itself is also simply performed.

In terms of hospitalization time, despite the fact that TEO has shown the smallest time, other authors also show very similar results. Some reports do not present this pattern because they described complicated cases, when long hospitalization was needed, and others because the follow up protocol demanded a longer hospitalization time.

The variable follow up after surgery, expressed in years (Graph XI) reflects the importance and the stability of the local excision surgeries. In several reports, the follow up time has been studied between 10 and 15 years. In our experience, the follow up time is in between 2 months and 8 years.

In this way, the challenge of idealizing, projecting and using a surgical endoscopic instrument of low costs, and adequate for its main purposes, i. e. appropriate for use in transanal endoscopic surgeries, was fully achieved.

The results of the TEO showed and discussed in the present study, compared to the international literature, demonstrated that the TEO is an adequate and feasible procedure for the local excision of rectal tumors.

5. Conclusions

1. The proctoscope specially designed and built for the TEO has shown appropriate, efficient and of low costs;
2. The TEO was easily performed on lesions of the mid and inferior third rectal tumors;
3. The results obtained with TEO were favorable and similar to those obtained with other available techniques for endoscopic transanal resection that are of high costs and of less availability.

6. References

[1] Balani A, Turoldo A, Braini A, Scaramucci M, Roseano M, Leggeri A. Local excision for rectal cancer. J Surg Oncol 2000; 74: 158-62.

[2] Nastro P, Beral D, Hartley J, Monson JR. Local excision of rectal cancer: review of literature. Dig Surg 2005; 22 (1-2): 6-15.

[3] Stipa S, Stipa F, Ziparo V. Tratamento cirúrgico de câncer de reto: Ressecção local. In: Rossi BM, Nakagawa WT, Ferreira FO, Aguiar Jr S, Lopes A . Câncer de Cólon, Reto e Anus. Ed. Tecmedd, 2005, p. 275.

[4] Kraske P. Zur exstirpation hochsitzender Mastdarmkrebse. Verh Dtsch Ges Chir 1884, 14: 464.

[5] Mason AY. Surgical access to the rectum: A transphincteric exposure. Proc R Soc Med 1970, 63(suppl): 91-4.

[6] Rothenberger DA, Garcia-Agüilar J. Role of local excision in the treatment of rectal câncer. Semin Surg Oncol 2000 ; 19(4): 367-75.

[7] Heintz A, Braunstein S, Menke H. Local excision of rectal tumors. Indications, preoperative diagnosis, surgical technique and results. Med Klin 1992; 87(5): 236-41.

[8] Buess GF. Local surgical treatment of rectal cancer. Eur J Cancer 1995; 31 A (7-8): 1233-7.

[9] Whitlow CB, Beck DE; Gathright JB. Surgical excision of large rectal villous adenomas. Surg Oncol Clin N Am 1996; 5(3): 723-34.

[10] Reid AJ - Echocolonoscopy - an indispensable procedure before and after transanal endoscopic microsurgery. Endosc Surg Allied Technol 1993; 1(1): 47-8.

[11] Graham RA, Hackford AW, Wazer DE. Local excision of rectal carcinoma: A safe alternative for more advanced tumors? J Surg Oncol 1999; 70: 235-8.

[12] Guerrieri M, Paganini A, Feliciotti F, Zenobi P, Lugnani F, Lezoche E. Echography in minimally invasive surgery. Ann Ital Chir 1999; 70(2): 211-5.

[13] Kneist W, Terzic A, Burghardt J, Heintz A, Junginger T. Selection of patients with rectal tumors for local excision based on preoperative diagnosis. Results of a consecutive evaluation study of 552 patients. Chirurgie, 2004 ; 75(2): 169-75.

[14] Glancy DG, Pullyblank AM, Thomas MG. The role of colonoscopic endoanal ultrasound scanning (EUS) in selecting patients suitable for resection by transanal endoscopic microsurgery (TEM). Colorectal Dis 2005; 7(2): 148-50.

[15] Biggers OR, Beart RW, Ilstrup DM. Local excision of rectal cancer. Dis Colon Rectum 1986; 29(6): 374-7.

[16] Budhoo M R & Hancock B Transanal excision of early rectal carcinoma - review of a personal series. Colorectal Dis 2000; 2 (2): 73-6.
[17] Koscinski T, Malinger S, Drews M. Local excision of rectal carcinoma not-exceeding the muscularis layer. Colorectal Dis 2003, 5 (2): 159-63.
[18] Beral DL, Monson JR. Is local excision of T2/T3 rectal cancers adequate?. Recent Results Cancer Res 2005; 165: 120-35.
[19] Guillem JG, Chessin DB, Jeong SY, Kim W, Fogarty JM. Contemporary applications of transanal endoscopic microsurgery: technical innovations and limitations. Clin Colorectal Cancer 2005; 5(4): 268-73.
[20] Aguilar JG, Mellgren A, Sirivongs P, Buie D, Madoff RD, Rothenberger DA. Local excision of rectal cancer without adjuvant therapy. A word of caution. Annals Surg. 2000; 231(3): 345-51.
[21] Buess G, Kipfmuller K, Naruhn M, Braunstein S, Junginger T. Endoscopic microsurgery of rectal tumors. Endoscopy 1987; 19 Suppl 1: 38-42.
[22] Buess G, Kipfmuller K, Hack D, Grussner R, Heintz A, Junginger T. Technique of transanal endoscopic microsurgery. Surg Endosc 1988; 2(2): 71-5.
[23] Swanstrom LL, Smiley P, Zelko J, Cagle L. Videoendoscopic transanal-rectal tumor excision. Am J Surg 1997; 173(5): 383-5.
[24] Yamashita Y, Sakai T, Maekawa T, Shirakusa T. Clinical use of a front lifting hood rectoscope tube for transanal endoscopic microsurgery. Surg Endosc 1998; 12(2): 151-3.
[25] Kakizoe S, Kakizoe K, Kakizoe Y, Kakizoe H, Kakizoe T, Kakizoe S. Rectal expander-assisted transanal endoscopic microsurgery in rectal tumors. Surg Laparosc Endosc 1998; 8(2): 117-9.
[26] Ikeda Y, Koyanagi N, Mori M, Akahoshi K, Ueyama T, Sugimachi K. Transanal endoscopic microsurgery for T1 rectal cancer in patients with synchronous colorectal cancer. Surg Endosc 1999; 13(7): 710-2.
[27] Hojo K, Koyama Y, Moriya Y. Lymphatic spread and its prognostic value in patients with rectal cancer. Am J Surg 1983; 144: 350-4.
[27] Leemis LM & Trivedi KS. A comparison of approximate interval estimator for the Bernoulli parameter. Am Statist. 1996, 50(1): 63-8.
[28] Jessup JM, Bothe A Jr, Stone MD. Preservation of sphincter function in rectal carcinoma by a multimodality treatment approach. Sur Oncol Clin North Am 1992; 1:137-45.
[29] Enker, WE, Paty PB, Minsky BD, Cohen AM. Restorative or preservative operations in the treatment of rectal cancer. Surg Oncol Clin North Am 1992; 1: 57-69.
[30] Fortunato L, Ahmad NR, Yeung RS, Coia LR, Eisenberg BL, Sigurdson ER, Yeh K, Weese JL, Hoffman JP. Long-term follow-up of local excision and radiation therapy for invasive rectal cancer. Dis Colon Rectum 1995; 38:1193-1199.
[31] Wind G, Nottberg H, Keller R, Schmid KW, Bunte H. Surgical cure for early rectal carcinomas (T1). Transanal endoscopic microsurgery vs anterior resection. Dis Colon Rectum 1996; 39 (9): 969-76.

[32] Heintz A, Morschel M, Junginger T. Comparison of results after transanal endoscopic microsurgery and radical resection for T1 carcinoma of the rectum. Surg Endosc 1998; 12(9): 1145-8.
[33] Lee W, Lee D, Choi S, Chun H. Transanal endoscopic microsurgery and radical surgery for T1 and T2 rectal cancer. Surg Endosc 2003; 17(8): 1283-7.
[34] Whiteway J et al. The role of surgical local excision in the treatment of rectal cancer. Br J Surg 1985, 72: 694-7.
[35] Morson BC, Bussey HJR, Samoorian S. Policy of local excision for early cancer of the colorectum. Gut 1977; 18: 1045-50.
[36] Stearns MW, Sternberg SS, DeCosse JJ. Treatment alternatives: localized rectal cancer. Cancer 1984; 54: 2691-4.
[37] Buess G. Review: transanal endoscopic microsurgery (TEM). J R Coll Surg Edinb 1983; 38 (4): 239-45.
[38] Buess G, Kipfmuller K, Ibald R, Heintz A, Hack D, Braunstein S, Gabbert H, Junginger T. Clinical results of transanal endoscopic microsurgery. Surg Endosc 1988; 2(4): 245-50.
[39] Nakagoe T, Hishikawa H, Sawai T, Tsuji T, Tanaka K, Ayabe H. Surgical technique and outcome of gasless video endoscopic transanal rectal tumour excision. Brit J Surg 2002; 89, 769-74.
[40] Coco C, Magistrelli P, Granone P, Roncolini G, Picciocchi A. Conservative surgery for early câncer of the distal rectum. Dis Colon Rectum 1992; 35: 131-6.
[41] Buess G, Kayser J. Technique and indications for sphincter-Saving transanal resection in rectal carcinoma. Buess G, Kayser J. Chir 1996; 67 (2): 121-8.
[42] Said S, Stippel D. 10 years experiences with transanal endoscopic microsurgery. Histopathologic and clinical analysis. Chirurg. 1996; 67(2): 139-44.
[43] Kipfmuller K, Buess G, Naruhn M, Junginger T. Training program for transanal endoscopaic microsurgery. Surg Endosc 1988; 2(1): 24-7.
[44] Spalinger R, Schlumpf R, Largiader F. Transanal endoscopic microsurgery - experiences at the Zurich University Hospital. Schweiz Rundsch Med Prax 1998; 87 (33): 1014-8.
[45] Demartines N, von Flue MO, Harder FH. Transanal endoscopaic microsurgical excision of rectal tumors: indications and results. World J Surg 2000; 25(7): 870-5.
[46] Buess GF, Raestrup H. Transanal endoscopic microsurgery. Surg Oncol Clin Am 2001; 10(3): 709-31.
[47] Lloyd GM, Sutton CD, Marshall LJ, Baragwanath P, Jameson JS, Scott AND. Transanal endoscopic microsurgery - lessons from a single UK centre series. Col Dis 2002; 4(6): 467-9.
[48] von Flue M, Harder F. Transanal endoscopic microsurgery (TEM): indications and limitations. Schweiz Med Wochenschr 1994; 124(41): 1800-6.
[49] Corman ML . Colon & Rectal Surgery. Fifth edition. Lippincott Williams & Wilkins, 2005.
[50] Guillem JG, Paty PB, Cohen AM. *Surgical treatment of colorectal cancer*. CA Cancer J Clin. 1997; 47: 113.

[51] Killingback M, Barron P, Dent OF . Local recurrence after curative resection of cancer of the rectum without total mesorectal excision. Dis Colon Rectum 2001; 44 (4): 473-86.

9

Diagnosis and Endoscopic Treatments of Rectal Varices

Takahiro Sato, Katsu Yamazaki and Jun Akaike
Department of Gastroenterology, Sapporo Kosei General Hospital, Sapporo
Japan

1. Introduction

Esophagogastric varices are considered to be the most common complication in patients with portal hypertension, while ectopic varices, that is, those outside of the esophagogastric region, are less common. Rectal varices represent portal systemic collaterals that are manifested as discrete dilated submucosal veins and constitute a pathway for portal venous flow between the superior rectal veins of the inferior mesenteric system and the middle inferior rectal veins of the iliac system. Rectal varices are an infrequent but potentially serious cause of hematochezia. Massive bleeding from rectal varices occurs rarely, with a frequency ranging from 0.5% to 3.6% (1-3). In this chapter, we describe the diagnostic modalities and endoscopic treatments for rectal varices in patients with portal hypertension.

2. Diagnosis of rectal varices

Endoscopy is the principal method for diagnosis of rectal varices. Endoscopic ultrasonography (EUS) can detect the presence and number of rectal varices better than endoscopy (4). Recently, color Doppler ultrasonography has allowed us to detect fine small blood flow (5). Sato et al. have reported the usefulness of percutaneous color Doppler ultrasonography (CDUS) for the hemodynamic evaluation of rectal varices (6).

Although endoscopic injection sclerotherapy (EIS) (7) and endoscopic band ligation (EBL) (8) for esophageal varices are well-established therapies, there is no standard treatment for rectal varices. In this article, we also review the therapeutic effects and complications of EIS versus EBL on rectal varices in patients with portal hypertension. Several diagnostic procedures have been performed to evaluate rectal varices, including endoscopy, magnetic resonance (MR) angiography, EUS. Endoscopy is the principal method for diagnosis of rectal varices and MR angiography is useful for evaluating the overall portosystemic collateral circulation. On the other hand, conventional EUS (7.5 or 12 MHz) reveals rectal varices as rounded, oval, or longitudinal echo-free structures in the submucosa and also shows perirectal veins outside the rectal wall (4,9,10). With endoscopic color Doppler ultrasonography (ECDUS), color flow images in blood vessels can be obtained, and ECDUS allows for more detailed observation of the hemodynamics of rectal varices than EUS (11). CDUS is a simpler, more non-invasive method than ECDUS and it enables us to detect slight blood flow and to evaluate the portal venous system. Nelson et al. concluded that CDUS was valuable for accurate determination of the direction of portal flow and patency of the vessel (12). Sato et al. have reported the usefulness of CDUS for the hemodynamic evaluation of rectal varices and compared velocities of rectal varices with CDUS and colonoscopic findings, and they concluded that CDUS was a useful noninvasive tool in the evaluation of portal hemodynamics, including the observation of blood flow in rectal varices (6).

2.1 Diagnosis of rectal varices via endoscopy

Endoscopy is the principal method for the diagnosis of rectal varices; it is a useful modality for diagnosing and observing rectal varices of a certain size and extent, and has a very sensitive predictive value for variceal hemorrhage. The endoscopic findings for rectal varices were evaluated according to the grading system outlined in 'The General Rules for Recording Endoscopic Findings of Esophago-gastric Varices 'prepared by the Japanese Research Committee on Portal Hypertension (13).

The form (F) of the varices was classified as small and straight (F_1), enlarged and tortuous (F_2), large and coil-shaped (F_3), or no varices after treatment (F_0). The fundamental color of the varices was classified as either white (Cw) or blue (Cb). The red color sign (RC) referred to dilated, small vessels or telangiectasia on the variceal surface. RC shows a high risk of variceal bleeding based on endoscopic findings (Table 1). The following images show: blue color and red color-positive coil-shaped rectal varices (Fig.1-a); blue color and red color-positive enlarged tortuous rectal varices (Fig.1-b), and a white plug on the rectal variceal surface in a patient with a case of rectal variceal bleeding (Fig.1-c).

Form (F)
F_1: small, straight
F_2: enlarged tortuous
F_3: coil-shaped
F_0: no varices after treatment
Fundamental color of the varices (C)
Cw: white
Cb: blue
Red color sign (RC): dilated, small vessels or telangiectasia on the variceal surface
RC_0: no RC sign
RC_1: only a few RC signs
RC_2: several RC signs
RC_3: many RC signs
Bleeding signs
Gushing bleeding
Spurting bleeding
Red plug
White plug
Mucosal finding
Erosion
Ulcer
Scar

Table 1. The General Rules for Recording Endoscopic Findings of Esophago-gastric Varices prepared by the Japanese Research Committee on Portal Hypertension

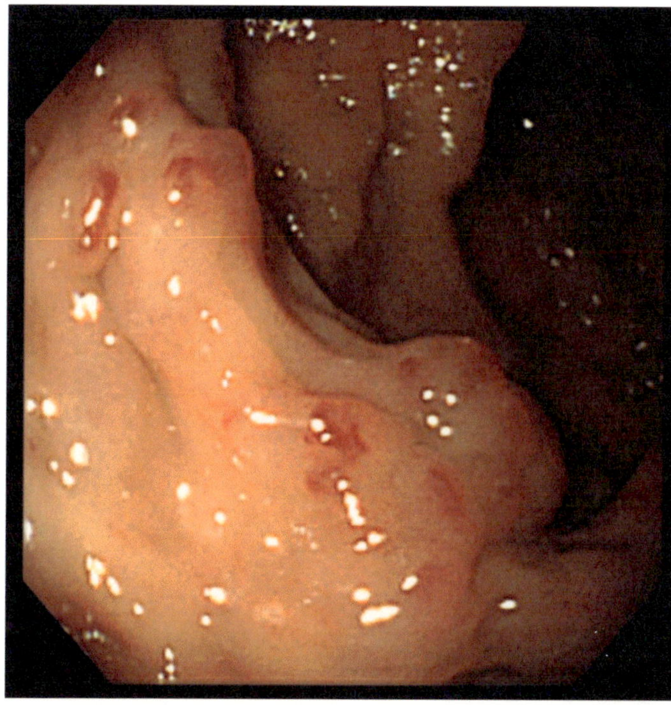

Fig. 1a. Endoscopy showing blue color and red color-positive coil-shaped rectal varices.

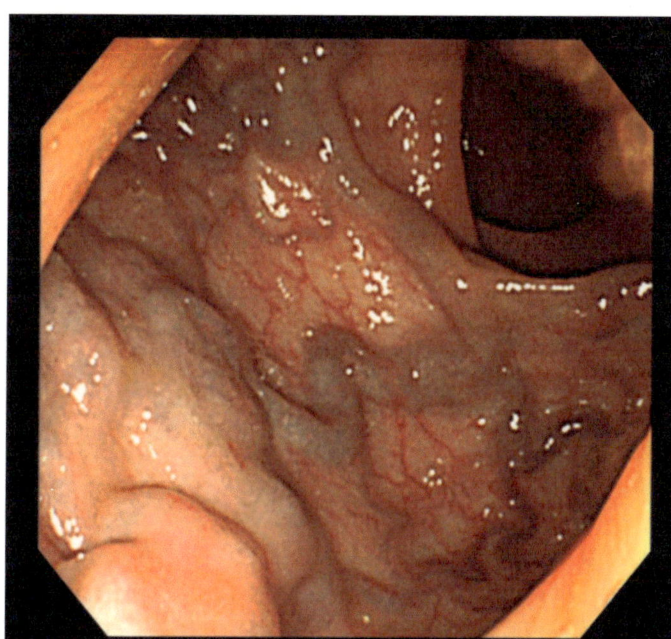

Fig. 1b. Endoscopy showing blue color and red color-positive enlarged tortuous rectal varices.

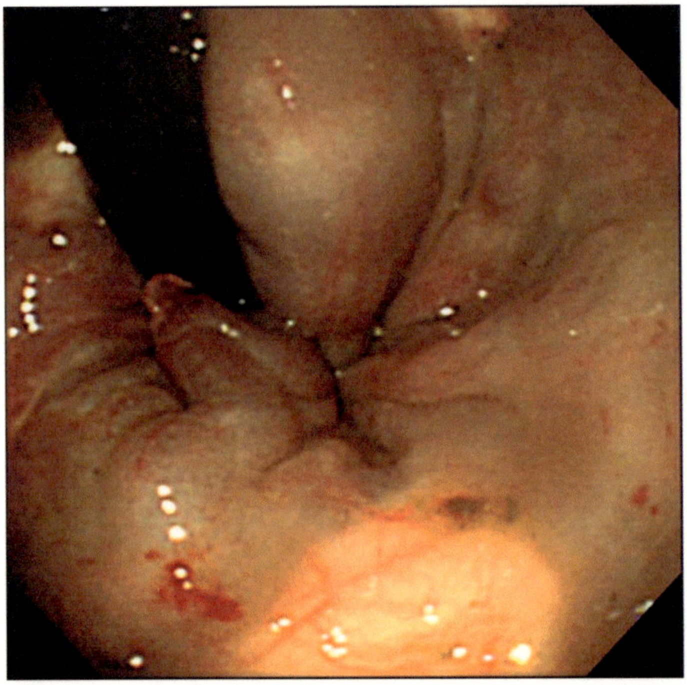

Fig. 1c. Endoscopy show a white plug on the rectal variceal surface in a patient with a case of rectal variceal bleeding.

Hemorrhoids are vascular cushions resulting from arteriolar venous communications in the hemorrhoidal plexus, with no direct communication with any of the major branches of the portal venous system being demonstrated. Fast-Fourier transform analysis of blood flow in the intramural rectal varices showed a continuous wave with a pulsatile wave in some patients. This phenomenon explains the coexistence of rectal varices and hemorrhoids, whereby blood from the hemorrhoids flows into the rectal varices at the anal site, causing a pulsatile blood flow wave from the hemorrhoids (arteriolar venous communication).

2.2 Diagnosis of rectal varices via endoscopic ultrasonography (EUS) and endoscopic color Doppler ultrasonography (ECDUS)

EUS has become a useful modality for hemodynamic diagnosis of esophagogastric varices (14,15). The usefulness of EUS (4,9,10) in the hemodynamic diagnosis of rectal varices has been described, and Dhiman et al. found rectal varices via endoscopy in 43% of patients and via EUS in 75% of patients with portal hypertension (10). Sato et al. demonstrated that intramural rectal varices, peri-rectal collateral veins, and the communicating veins between intramural rectal varices and peri-rectal collateral veins could be observed clearly via an ultrasonic microprobe (16). ECDUS is better equipped than conventional EUS to visualize in detail the hemodynamics of esophagogastric varices (17,18). With ECDUS, color flow images in blood vessels can be obtained, and ECDUS allows for more detailed observation of the hemodynamics of rectal varices than EUS (11). ECDUS is useful for detecting rectal varices through color flow images, and it is a necessary tool for effective and safe EIS by calculating the velocity of blood flow in rectal varices (Fig.2).

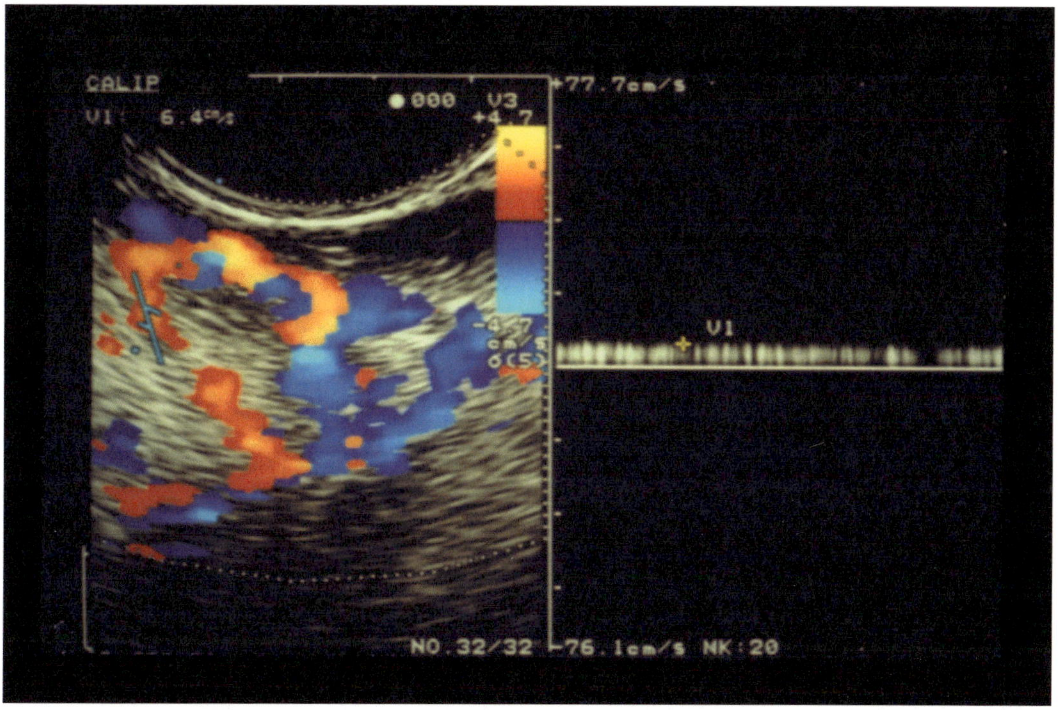

Fig. 2. Color flow images of rectal varices and inflowing vessel with endoscopic color Doppler ultrasonography

2.3 Diagnosis of rectal varices via percutaneous color Doppler ultrasonography (CDUS)

Recently, color Doppler ultrasonography has become widely accepted for the assessment of the hemodynamics of abdominal vascular systems, but few color Doppler findings of gastrointestinal varices have been reported. Komatsuda et al. reported the usefulness of CDUS for the diagnosis of gastric and duodenal varices (19), and Sato et al. concluded that CDUS was useful for evaluating the hemodynamics of gastric varices (20). CDUS cannot be performed successfully without a suitable acoustic window. Impediments such as bowel gas, body habitus, and cirrhosis limit the value of sonography for assessing the portal venous system. In addition, with color Doppler sonography, it is difficult to observe the collateral veins situated far from the probe due to the limitations of Doppler sensitivity. The rectal wall was detected at the back area of the vagina in females or prostate in males by sonography and rectal varices could be observed through the bladder filled with urine via color Doppler ultrasonography (Fig.3).

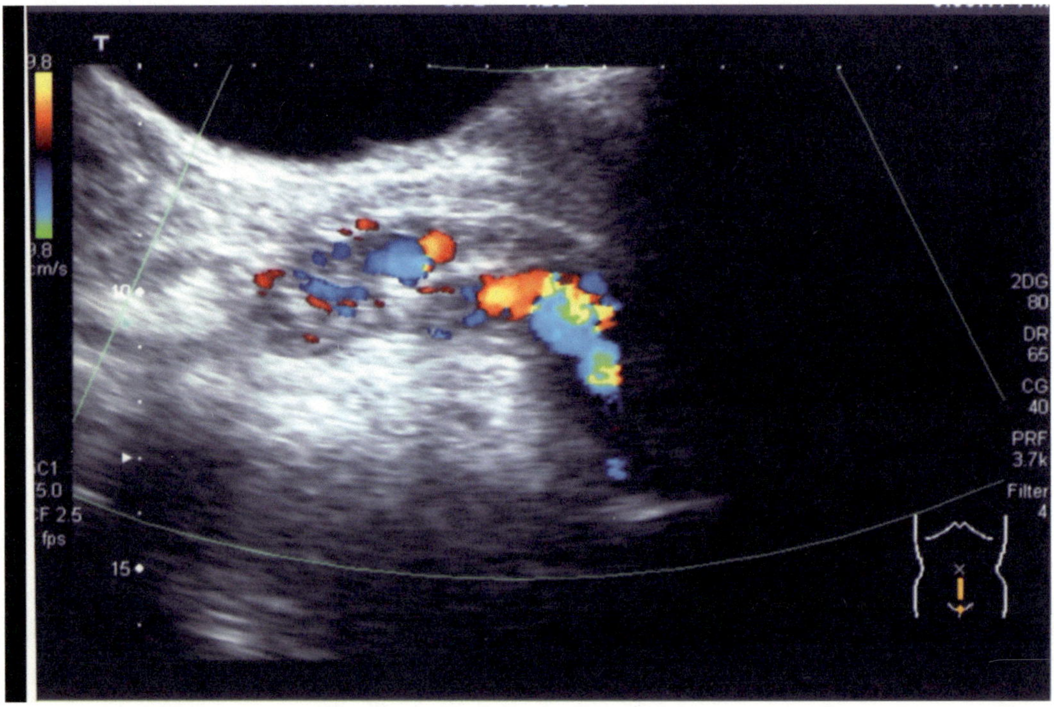

Fig. 3. Color flow images of rectal varices with color Doppler ultrasonography.

Sato et al. compared the velocities of rectal varices with CDUS and colonoscopic findings (6). The majority of the 44 cases underwent colonoscopy after diagnosis with color Doppler. In this study, the mean velocity of the F2 type rectal varices was significantly higher than that of the F1 type, and the mean velocity of the RC-positive varices was significantly higher than that of RC-negative varices with color Doppler ultrasonography. These results suggest that the measurement of velocity in rectal varices via color Doppler ultrasonography is useful in diagnosing the grade of rectal varices. CDUS is a useful noninvasive tool in the evaluation of portal hemodynamics, including the observation of blood flow in rectal varices.

3. Endoscopic treatments of rectal varices

Rectal varices are considered to occur infrequently, however, several articles have reported that they occur with high frequency in patients with hepatic abnormalities (21-23). Hosking et al. reported that 44 % of 100 consecutive cirrhotic patients had anorectal varices (21). Other studies found that the prevalence of anorectal varices was 78% in 72 portal hypertensive patients (22) and 43% in 103 cirrhotic patients (23). Although EIS and EBL for esophageal varices are well-established therapies, there is no standard treatment for rectal varices.

Various medical treatments have been used to control bleeding from rectal varices, but none of these is currently considered to be a standard method. Surgical approaches include portosystemic shunting, ligation, and under-running suturing (21). Some investigators have reported that interventional radiologic techniques such as transjugular intrahepatic portosystemic shunts were successfully employed for rectal variceal bleeding (24-26). Several cases of successful treatment of rectal varices with endoscopic treatments have been reported. Wang et al. first reported the usefulness of EIS in treating rectal varices and found it to be effective for controlling bleeding (27). EBL was introduced as a new method for treating esophageal varices, and it is reportedly both easier to perform and safer than EIS. Several cases of successful treatment of rectal varices using EBL have been reported (28-30).

3.1 EIS for rectal varices

We performed EIS in 21 of the 30 patients, who were successfully treated without complications. EIS was performed using 5% ethanolamine oleate with iopamidol (5%EOI), which was injected intermittently under fluoroscopy. The procedure was performed using a flexible GI endoscope (GIF XQ200; Olympus Optical Co., Ltd., Tokyo, Japan) by a free-hand method, using a 25-gauge injection needle. EIS was repeated every week until the disappearance of all rectal varices and RC signs were confirmed by endoscopy. Fluoroscopic observation with infusion of 5%EOI was performed to determine the extent of the varices, taking care that 5%EOI did not flow into the systemic circulation. We decided the amount of 5%EOI on depiction of passageways (superior rectal vein) of rectal varices. After EIS, colonoscopy revealed shrinkage of the rectal varices in all 21 patients, with no complications reported.

It is necessary to evaluate the hemodynamics of the rectal varices before EIS to avoid severe complications such as pulmonary embolism, and the sclerosant should be injected slowly under fluoroscopy (Fig.4).

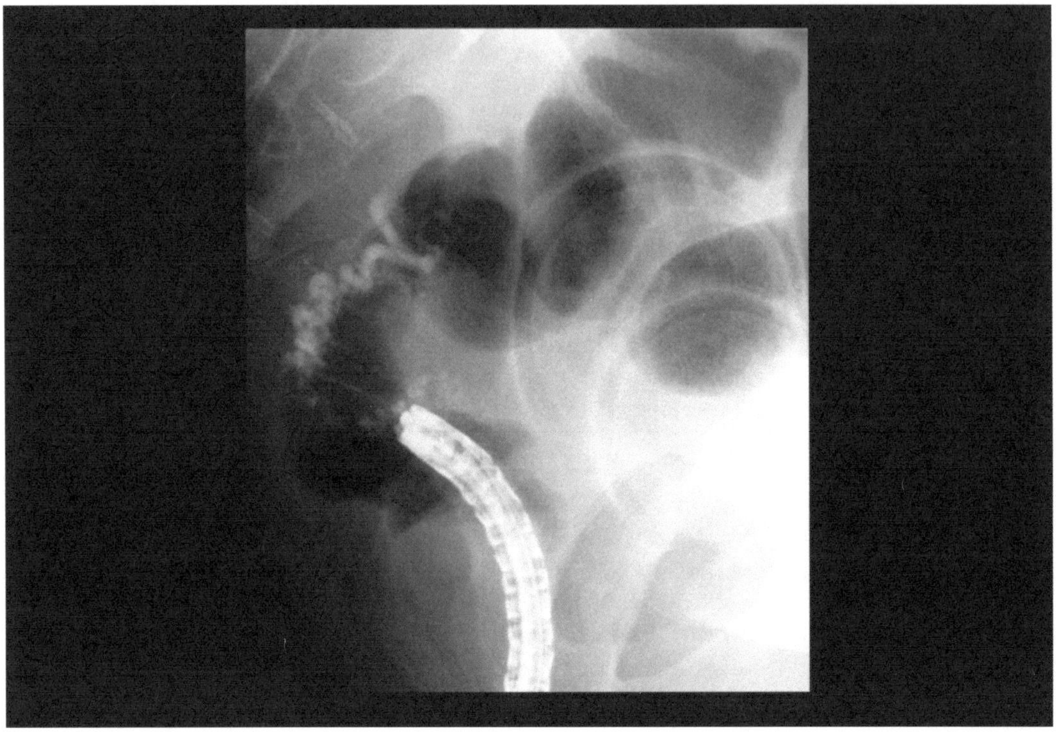

Fig. 4. Fluoroscopic observation with infusion of 5%EOI was performed.

3.2 EBL for rectal varices

EBL was introduced as a new method for treating esophageal varices, and it is reportedly both easier to perform and safer than EIS. Several cases of successful treatment of rectal varices using EBL have been reported. Levine et al. treated rectal varices initially with EIS, and 1 week later, EBL was performed on the remaining rectal varices (28). These investigators described EBL as a safe and effective therapy for rectal varices (30).

EBL was performed in 9 patients on our ward; it was performed weekly using a pneumo-activated EBL device (Sumitomo Bakelite, Tokyo, Japan), and bands were placed on the varices. An overtube was not used during EBL (Fig.5). After EBL, colonoscopy revealed ulcers and improvement of the varices in the rectum of all 9 patients. Eight of the 9 patients experienced no operative complications. However, colonoscopy revealed bleeding from ulcers after EBL in 1 case, in whom endoscopic clipping was performed on the oozing ulcers.

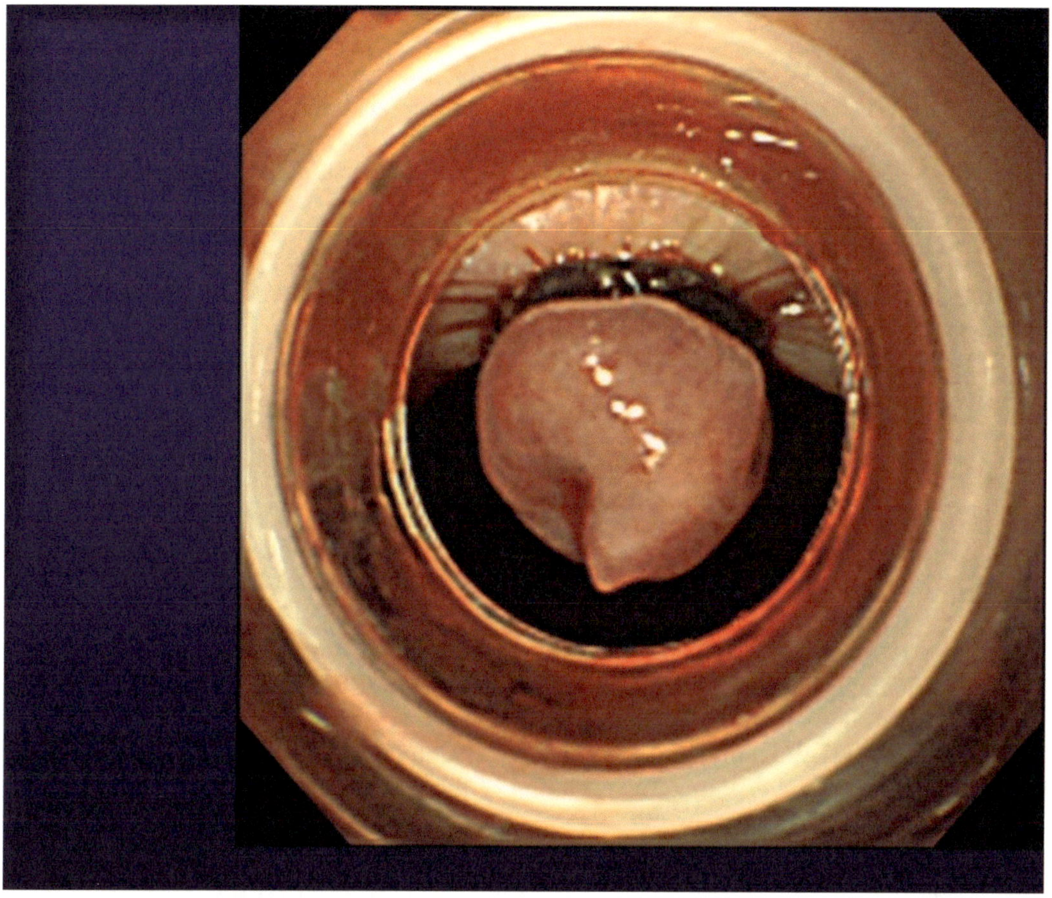

Fig. 5. EBL was performed weekly using a pneumo-activated EBL device.

3.3 Comparison EIS and EBL for rectal varices

We have used EIS or EBL to treat rectal varices. In our ward, we retrospectively evaluated the therapeutic effects and rates of recurrence of rectal varices after EIS or EBL. We performed EIS in 21 of the 30 patients, who were successfully treated without complications. The overall recurrence rate for rectal varices over the 1-year follow-up period after treatments was 10 of 24 (41.7%). The patients with recurrence included 5 of the 15 patients (33.3%) receiving EIS and 5 of the 9 (55.6%) who received EBL. The recurrence rate was not significantly different between the EIS group and EBL groups, although recurrence tended to be more frequent with EBL.

EBL may be suitable as an initial treatment for rectal varices, but it appears that the varices can easily recur after EBL (31,32). The recurrence rate for bleeding in the EBL group was significantly higher than in the EIS group in our result. All four patients with recurrence of bleeding had been treated using EBL.

EIS appears to be superior to EBL with regard to long-term effectiveness and complications following endoscopic treatment of rectal varices in patients with portal hypertension. More investigations are necessary in larger numbers of patients before evidence-based treatment recommendations can be made.

4. Conclusion

Hemorrhage from rectal varices should be kept in mind in patients with portal hypertension presenting with lower gastrointestinal bleeding. It is difficult to determine the best treatment strategy for rectal varices because of inaccessibility, initial difficulty in diagnosis and subsequent difficulty in treatment.

5. Acknowledgment

The authors thank Dr Jouji Toyota, Dr Yoshiyasu Karino, Dr Takumi Ohmura of Sapporo Kosei Hospital, for their help with the manuscript.

6. References

[1] McCormack TT, Bailey HR, Simms JM, Johnson AG. (1984). Rectal varices are not piles. *Br J Surg* 71:163.

[2] Johansen K, Bardin J, Orloff MJ. (1980). Massive bleeding from hemorrhoidal varices in portal hypertension. *JAMA* 224:2084-5.

[3] Wilson SE, Stone RT, Christie JP, Passaro E. (1979). Massive lower gastrointestinal bleeding from intestinal varices. *Arch Surg* 114:1158-61.

[4] Dhiman RK, Choudhuri G, Saraswat VA, et al. (1993). Endoscopic ultrasonographic evaluation of the rectum in cirrhotic portal hypertension. *Gastrointest Endosc* 39:635-40.

[5] Ueno N, Sasaki A, Tomiyama T, et al. (1997). Color Doppler ultrasonography in the diagnosis of cavernous transformation of the portal vein. *J Clin Ultrasound* 25:227-33.

[6] Sato T, Yamazaki K, Toyota J, Karino Y, Ohmura T, Akaike J. (2007). Diagnosis of rectal varices via color Doppler ultrasonography. *Am J Gastroenterol* 102:2253-8.

[7] The Veterans Affairs Cooperative Variceal Sclerotherapy Group. (1991). Prophylactic sclerotherapy for esophageal varices in men with alcoholic liver disease. *N Engl J Med* 324:1779-84.

[8] Goff GV, Reveille RM, Stiegmann GV. (1988). Endoscopic sclerotherapy versus endoscopic variceal ligation: esophageal symptoms, complications and motility. *Am J Gastroenterol* 83:1240-4.

[9] Yachha SK, Dhiman RK, Gupta R, et al. (1993). Endosonographic evaluation of the rectum in children with extrahepatic portal venous obstruction. *J Pediatr Gastroenterol Nutr* 23:438-41.

[10] Dhiman RK, Saraswat VA, Choudhuri G, Sharma BC, Pandey R, Naik SR. (1999). Endosonographic, endoscopic, and histologic evaluation of alterations in the rectal venous system in patients with portal hypertension. *Gastrointest Endosc* 49:218-27.

[11] Sato T, Yamazaki K, Akaike J. (2006). Evaluation of the hemodynamics of rectal varices by endoscopic ultrasonography. *J Gastroenterol* 41:588-92.

[12] Nelson RC, Lovett KE, Chezmar JL, et al. (1987). Comparison of pulsed Doppler sonography and angiography in patients with portal hypertension. *Am J Roentgenol* 149:77-81.